Stroke in Practice

Stroke in Practice

FROM DIAGNOSIS TO EVIDENCE-BASED MANAGEMENT

CHRISTOS TZIOTZIOS

BA, MA, MB, BChir (Cantab)
Core Medical Trainee
Cambridge University Hospitals

JESSE DAWSON

BSc, MBChB, MRCP, MD
Clinical Lecturer in Clinical Pharmacology and Stroke
University of Glasgow

and

MATTHEW WALTERS

MBChB, MSc, FRCP, MD
Professor of Clinical Pharmacology
University of Glasgow

Foreword by

Kennedy R Lees

BSc, MBChB, FRCP, MD
Professor of Cerebrovascular Medicine
University of Glasgow
Secretary General, European Stroke Organisation

Radcliffe Publishing
London • New York

Radcliffe Publishing Ltd
33–41 Dallington Street
London
EC1V 0BB
United Kingdom

www.radcliffepublishing.com

Electronic catalogue and worldwide online ordering facility.

British Library Cataloguing in Publication Data

A catalogue record for this book is available from the British Library.

ISBN-13: 978 184619 473 3

The paper used for the text pages of this book is FSC certified. FSC (The Forest Stewardship Council) is an international network to promote responsible management of the world's forests.

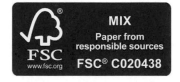

Typeset by KnowledgeWorks Global Ltd, Chennai, India
Printed and bound by Hobbs the Printers, Totton, Hampshire, UK

Contents

Foreword

In recent years, stroke has transformed from a Cinderella condition into a high priority for clinicians and healthcare systems. It is no longer the province of a few neurologists or rehabilitationists. Stroke specialists have skills encompassing emergency medicine, neurological diagnosis, cardiovascular, internal medicine, and rehabilitation topics. The treatable nature of the acute presentation and the urgency yet simplicity of intervention with thrombolysis dictates that diagnosis and immediate care must be delivered by clinicians from many backgrounds. The diversity of presentations, the real if uncommon risks of treatment, and the subtleties of acute imaging findings mandate that most medical and nursing staff should be familiar with common issues in practical stroke management. This text is written by clinicians with experience of stroke management in a practical setting, working with facilities available in typical general hospitals. It is directed at the non-specialist and emphasises practicality over academic niceties. If it inspires enthusiasm for a fascinating condition and convinces the reader that stroke is preventable, treatable, and yet potentially devastating for patients and their families, it will justify its existence.

Professor Kennedy R Lees
Professor of Cerebrovascular Medicine
University of Glasgow
Secretary General, European Stroke Organisation
April 2011

About the authors

Dr Christos Tziotzios BA, MA, MB, BChir (Cantab)
Christos Tziotzios is currently a Core Medical Trainee at Cambridge University Hospitals. He read medicine at the University of Cambridge, where he also engaged in teaching and research. His prior academic and research background is in basic and clinical pharmacology. He developed an interest in stroke medicine in the capacity of Honorary Clinical Fellow at the University of Glasgow.

Dr Jesse Dawson BSc, MBChB, MRCP, MD
Jesse Dawson is a clinical lecturer in clinical pharmacology and stroke at the University of Glasgow whose main interests are prevention of stroke, with particular emphasis on novel therapies. He is a graduate of the University of Glasgow and trained in the Acute Stroke Unit at the Western Infirmary.

Professor Matthew Walters MBChB, MSc, FRCP, MD
Matthew Walters is professor of clinical pharmacology at the University of Glasgow and an honorary consultant physician at the Acute Stroke Unit of the city's Western Infirmary. He is lead clinician for stroke in West Glasgow and director of the Scottish Stroke Research Network.

To my lovely wife Dimitra
CT

CHAPTER 1

Introduction

DEFINITIONS

A widely used definition of stroke is the *abrupt onset of a focal or global neurological deficit with no apparent cause other than vascular origin.*[1] The term covers a heterogeneous group of such vascular disorders, all with the potential to cause devastating neurological damage.[2]

The onset of stroke is *sudden* (usually over minutes) and can be either haemorrhagic or ischaemic. In ischaemia, the cessation of blood supply causes hypoxia and neuroglycopenia and subsequent energy failure. In haemorrhagic stroke, bleeding into the brain parenchyma occurs and causes neuronal damage via several mechanisms. Commonly seen *deficits* include dysphasia, dysarthria, hemianopia, motor weakness, ataxia, sensory loss, and neglect, but their expression is highly variable due to the complexity of brain anatomy and its vascular supply. Consciousness tends to be preserved and symptoms and signs manifest in a unilateral fashion. However, while the vast majority of deficits are focal, they can occasionally be more global.

In the medical literature, the term *stroke* is reserved for neurological deficits lasting more than 24 hours, and indeed the WHO definition sets this arbitrary time window as a prerequisite for distinguishing stroke from a *transient ischaemic attack* (TIA). The latter typically lasts less than 20 minutes but by definition no longer than 24 hours, with full recovery. Stroke and TIA should best be thought of as a continuum, as the same risk factors underpin both disease processes and the latter often heralds the former. The temporal threshold that separates stroke from TIA has been criticised and alternate definitions have been proposed; these are discussed in Chapter 7. *Cerebrovascular disease* is a broader term embracing stroke, vascular dementia, asymptomatic disorders of cerebral vessels, and TIA. It denotes a wide spectrum of disease caused by disturbances of cerebral blood flow or blood vessel pathology.[3]

EPIDEMIOLOGY

Stroke ranks as the third leading cause of death worldwide[4] and in the UK, where it ranks after heart disease and cancer. It is the second most common cause of lost disability-adjusted life years in high-income countries after ischaemic heart disease.[5, 6]

The incidence of stroke varies among countries and increases exponentially with age, as does the likelihood of a poor outcome after a cerebrovascular event. Stroke will therefore remain at the centre of national health statistics in our ageing society.[7]

It is estimated that 30-day case fatality rates for ischaemic stroke in Western societies range between 10 and 17%.[8] The likelihood of a poor outcome increases with stroke severity, either in terms of lesion size or the clinical deficit. Mortality in the first month after stroke has been reported to range from 2.5% in patients with lacunar infarcts[9] to 78% in patients with space-occupying hemispheric infarction.[10]

It has been argued that stroke causes a greater burden of disability than any other chronic disease,[11] and it comes as no surprise that the direct cost of stroke to the NHS in the UK is huge, estimated at £2.8 billion per year. Again, these direct NHS and total societal costs of stroke will rise steadily as the population ages.[12]

Focal cerebral ischaemia due to arterial occlusion accounts for the majority of strokes with some 80% of strokes in Western societies being of ischaemic aetiology, whereas haemorrhages account for the remaining 20%.[7] This balance differs between ethnic groups; however, on a worldwide scale, the majority of strokes are ischaemic.

OBJECTIVES OF THIS BOOK

The aim of this handbook is to provide an overview of *stroke* as a disease entity and a concise but analytical account of assessment and management strategies.

Having outlined some essential definitions and having demonstrated the burden of stroke, we will review the essential neuroanatomy and pathophysiology before considering stroke classification systems. Stroke syndromes, assessment of the suspected stroke patient, evidence-based management strategies, stroke mimics, stroke in the young adult, transient ischaemic attacks, and the role of different imaging strategies are then discussed in more detail.

REFERENCES

1. Smith WS. Cerebrovascular disease. In: *Harrison's Principles of Internal Medicine*. 17th international ed. McGraw-Hill Medical; 2008.
2. Zivin J. Approach to cerebrovascular disease. In: Goldman L, Ausiello D, editors. *Cecil Textbook of Medicine*. 22nd international ed. Saunders; 2004.
3. Kumar V, Abbas AK, Fausto N. *Robins and Cotran Pathologic Basis of Disease*. 7th international ed. Elsevier Saunders; 2004.

4. Warlow C, van Gijin J, Dennis M, *et al*. *Stroke: Practical Management*. 3rd ed. Blackwell; 2008.
5. Lopez AS, Mathers CD, Ezzati M, *et al*. Global and regional burden of disease and risk factors, 2001: systematic analysis of population health data. *Lancet*. 2006; **367**: 1747–57.
6. *Scottish Stroke Care Audit 2008 National Report*. Available at: www.strokeaudit.scot. nhs.uk/ (accessed June 2010).
7. Broderick JP, Adams HP, Barsan W, *et al*. Guidelines for the management of spontaneous intracerebral haemorrhage: a statement for healthcare professionals from a special writing group of the Stroke Council, American Heart Association. *Stroke* 1999; **30**: 905–15.
8. Feigin VL, Lawes CM, Bennett DA, *et al*. Stroke epidemiology: a review of population-based studies of incidence, prevalence and case-fatality in the late 20th century. *Lancet Neurol*. 2003; **2**: 43–53.
9. Norving B. Long-term prognosis after lacunar infarction. *Lancet Neurol*. 2003; **2**: 238–45.
10. Hacke W, Schwab S, Horn M, *et al*. 'Malignant' middle cerebral artery infarction: clinical course and prognostic signs. *Arch Neurol*. 1996; **53**: 309–15.
11. Adamson J, Beswick A, Ebrahim S. Stroke and disability. *Journal of Stroke and Cerebrovascular Diseases*. 2004; **13**(4).
12. National Audit Office. *Reducing Brain Damage: Faster access to better stroke care*. National Audit Office; 2005.

CHAPTER 2

Pathobiology, aetiology, and genetics

ISCHAEMIC STROKE
Pathophysiology

Cerebral ischaemia can be focal, usually caused by occlusion of a carotid, vertebral, or intracranial vessel, or global, usually as a consequence of failure of blood or oxygen supply to the whole brain. This typically follows profound hypotension or hypoxia. Following focal vascular occlusion, the extent of blood flow reduction depends on collateral blood flow, which is in turn dependent upon the site of occlusion, anatomy of the local vasculature, and duration of cerebral ischaemia. Infarction (death of brain tissue) occurs within four to 10 minutes from complete cessation of blood flow. When cerebral blood flow falls to approximately half the usual value (i.e., from 50 to about 20 mL/100 g tissue per minute), ischaemia without infarction results, and the affected brain remains viable unless this reduction in blood flow is prolonged for several hours or days. More minor degrees of ischaemia can however produce irreversible damage to highly vulnerable neurons. Restoration of blood flow prior to significant cell death may render symptoms to be transient, and this process is thought to be responsible for transient ischaemic attacks (TIAs). The central ischaemic zone is surrounded by a rim of tissue that is ischaemic but reversibly dysfunctional and is referred to as ischaemic penumbra. The ischaemic penumbra is a key concept in the treatment of stroke. As it remains viable for longer than the ischaemic core and can potentially be salvaged, it is an important therapeutic target for acute stroke treatments such as thrombolysis.[1]

In severe ischaemia, neurons are starved of oxygen and glucose, which subsequently causes mitochondrial failure and thus lack of ATP, the cell energy fuel. Depletion of these energy-rich compounds ensues within minutes and energy-dependent cell membrane pumps malfunction. This causes depolarisation of neuronal and glial cell membranes and allows the influx of calcium. Depolarisation of presynaptic terminals causes release of excitatory neurotransmitters, such as

TABLE 2.1 Causes of ischaemic stroke

Common	*Less common*
Thrombosis	Hypercoagulable disorders (such as protein C deficiency, antithrombin deficiency, protein S deficiency, thrombotic thrombocytopenic purpura, polycythaemia rubra vera, malignancy, nephritic syndrome, and SLE)
Embolic (e.g., due to atrial fibrillation, mural thrombus or septal aneurysms, paradoxical emboli, arterial dissection)	Vasculitis (such as Wegener's, PAN, Takayasu's, syphilitic, giant cell arteritis)

glutamate, which elevate metabolic demand at a time of inadequate supply and thus exacerbate cell injury. Neuronal calcium influx is further increased by a stimulatory effect on postsynaptic glutamate receptors. Lipid degradation and mitochondrial dysfunction leads to free radical production, the damaging effects of which adversely affect and severely disrupt cellular functions. Neuroprotective strategies aim to favourably alter these damaging cascades, and research in this field is ongoing. Further, it is known that pyrexia and hyperglycaemia may augment these processes, and control of these parameters may help limit neurological injury.[2]

Cerebral oedema may also follow an ischaemic stroke, and oedema may add to the neurological damage and injury.[3]

Aetiology

Aetiology does not influence the hyperacute management of ischaemic stroke, but establishing a cause is essential in order to reduce or prevent recurrence. History, examination, and baseline investigations are invaluable in narrowing the aetiological spectrum. A list of common and uncommon causes of ischaemic stroke is presented in Table 2.1.

Pathogenesis
Atherosclerosis

Atherosclerosis ranks first among the disorders leading to stroke and TIA. This can occur by way of in situ thrombosis at the site of an atherosclerotic lesion or via distal embolism of thrombus. This typically follows plaque ulceration and rupture but can arise due to haemorrhage into a plaque. The extent of brain tissue damage can depend on the speed of onset of the arterial obstruction. For example, if a patient develops gradual occlusion of a cerebral artery, collateral circulation and adaptation at the molecular level may occur and protect from damage in the event of complete arterial occlusion—so-called ischaemic preconditioning.

The roughened surface of an atherosclerotic plaque is frequently associated with platelet-fibrin thrombus formation, which is prone to breaking off and distal lodging in a smaller branch in a so-called *artery-to-artery embolisation*. In such cases, symptoms tend to be less dramatic than mainstem or larger vessel occlusion due to the less extensive territory affected. However, emboli are likely to cause symptoms as these distal arteries are end arteries that lack the potential for collateral flow. Intravascular thrombosis is frequently seen at foci of turbulent blood flow, such as at the bifurcation of the common carotid artery, the origin of the vertebral arteries, and the base of the aorta.

Cardioembolism

Emboli of cardiac origin can arise as a consequence of structural cardiac abnormalities or arrhythmias and commonly lodge in the cerebral circulation.

Mural thrombi

A dyskinetic segment of myocardium (such as that occurring following myocardial infarction) predisposes to mural thrombus formation, with anterior wall infarction being associated with the highest risk. Severe heart failure and cardiomyopathy are also associated with myocardial dyskinesia that promotes mural thrombi.

Valvular heart disease

Rheumatic heart disease and infective endocarditis, whether acute or subacute, are associated with systemic emboli. Non-bacterial and Libman-Sacks endocarditis may also cause cerebral emboli.

Mechanical prosthetic valves are associated with a higher incidence of ischaemic emboli than tissue valves and the risk is not completely abolished by oral anticoagulation. The overall incidence of stroke is 1–5% per year in patients with prosthetic heart valves despite anticoagulation.

Arrhythmias

Atrial fibrillation accounts for some 15% all ischaemic cerebrovascular events with the majority being due to emboli from left atrial mural thrombi. Amongst other factors, concurrent chronic hypertension, diabetes mellitus, and increasing age increases this risk. Embolism may accompany cardioversion, and the risk is higher shortly after development of atrial fibrillation.

Paradoxical emboli

A cardiac defect, such as patent foramen ovale (PFO), an atrial septal defect, or an arteriovenous malformation can allow entry of embolic material of venous origin to the arterial circulation. A PFO is seen in some 40% of patients with ischaemic events of unknown cause, and paradoxical emboli are assumed to be the underlying mechanism. The risk is increased in patients with concurrent atrial septal aneurysm and PFO.[4] Thrombus can also form at the site of a septal defect and subsequently embolise.

TABLE 2.2 Modifiable risk factors for stroke and risk reduction with treatments

Risk factor
Hypertension
Atrial fibrillation
Diabetes
Smoking
Hyperlipidaemia
Asymptomatic carotid stenosis
Carotid stenosis

Risk factors

A number of modifiable risk factors have been identified, and their control is key to reducing the incidence of stroke. An account of these is given in Table 2.2.

HAEMORRHAGIC STROKE

Pathophysiology

Subarachnoid haemorrhage, whether from a vascular malformation or berry aneurysm rupture, causes meningeal inflammation and subsequent vasospasm. The latter may result in cerebral ischaemia and brain tissue death by similar means to thrombotic occlusion.

Primary intraparenchymal haemorrhage causes infarction of the territory distal to the rupture through pressure effect and the toxic effects of blood breakdown products. The extravascular presence of blood implies an increase in total brain volume and a subsequent rise in intracranial pressure. This rise in intracranial pressure and cerebral oedema can cause significant neurological damage and may even cause cerebral herniation syndromes that result in brainstem damage and respiratory arrest.

Aetiology

Intracranial haemorrhages can be intraparenchymal, subarachnoid, or mixed, and a number of causes exist, the most common of which are presented in Table 2.3.

Risk factors

Hypertension is the single most important risk factor for intracerebral haemorrhage, especially in people younger than 55 years.

The risk of intracerebral haemorrhage is also increased by excessive alcohol consumption. Hypercholesterolaemia is less well established as a risk factor and some

TABLE 2.3 Causes of intracranial haemorrhage

Cause	Characteristics
Hypertension	Typical sites include the putamen, globus pallidus, thalamus, cerebellum, and pons. These areas are affected by a small vessel arteriopathy in chronic hypertension.
Haemorrhagic transformation of ischaemic infarct	Occurs frequently in ischaemic strokes (especially extensive lesions) and may involve basal ganglia, subcortical regions, and lobes.
Head trauma	Usually intraparenchymal in location.
Aneurysm	Subarachnoid, intraparenchymal, rarely subdural.
Metastatic lesions	More commonly with lung, melanoma, renal cell carcinoma, and thyroid; lobar involvement is common.
Coagulopathy	Relatively uncommon and may involve any region.
Amyloid angiopathy	Afflicts mainly the elderly and is a degenerative disease of brain vasculature; haemorrhage typically affects cortical areas.
Drugs	Seen with drugs such as amphetamine and cocaine and may be lobar or subarachnoid in location.

evidence suggests that risk of cerebral haemorrhage is increased with lower levels of serum cholesterol and with cholesterol-lowering therapy.

Haematological disorders, including haemophilia, clotting disorders are also associated with increased risk, as are iatrogenic causes such as anticoagulation with warfarin.

STROKE GENETICS

There is ample epidemiological evidence of a genetic predisposition to stroke. There are rare types of stroke that are monogenic (single gene) and follow a Mendelian pattern of inheritance. A representative number of such rare entities are presented in Table 2.4. Aspects of this topic will be further discussed in Chapter 9.

More commonly, stroke is polygenic and aetiology is multifactorial. Nevertheless, it is evident from twin and familial aggregation studies that predisposition to stroke is to some extent genetically determined.[5-7] Recent genome-wide association studies have identified a genetic locus on chromosome 12p13 to be associated (but not causally related) with total, ischaemic, and atherothrombotic stroke in white subjects.[8] Gene therapy for stroke remains remote from current clinical practice but gene markers may allow more effective screening and risk profiling and may play a role in the prevention and investigation of stroke in the future.

TABLE 2.4 Monogenic rare stroke

Clinical entity	Genetic culprit	Comments
CADASIL	NOTCH3	Cerebral autosomal dominant arteriopathy with subcortical infarcts and leukoencephalopathy.
MELAS	Multiple mitochondrial	Mitochondrial myopathy, encephalopathy, lactic acidosis, and stroke-like episodes. Seizures, recurrent headaches, and sensorineural deafness are also features. Onset of stroke episodes is usually before 40 years of age.
Ehlers-Danlos	COL3A1	Reduced levels of or faulty collagen, affecting joints, skin, and blood vessels; results in the characteristic joint hypermobility, hyperelastic skin, and fragile vessels often involved with rupture, aneurysm, or dissection.
Marfan's syndrome	FBN1	Aortic/cervical dissection in association with skeletal, cardiovascular, eye, and neurological abnormalities.
Fabry's disease	GAL	Alpha-galactosidase A deficiency leading to glycolipid accumulation in blood vessels and other organs; clinical manifestations include stroke as well as renal, cardiac, ocular, and dermatological complications.
Sickle-cell disease	HBB	Abnormally sickle-shaped red cells leading to vaso-occlusion by blood vessel narrowing causing cerebral infarction, among other complications.
Homocystinuria	CBS	Accumulation of homocysteine due to a defect in methionine metabolism and leading to multisystem manifestations, including premature atherosclerosis and stroke.

REFERENCES

1. Smith WS, Johnston SC, Easton D. Cerebrovascular diseases. In: *Harrison's Principles of Internal Medicine*. 17th international ed. McGraw-Hill; 2008.
2. Kunitz SC, Gross CRE, Heyman A, *et al*. The Pilot Stroke Data Bank: definition, design, and data. *Stroke*. 1984; **15**: 740–6.
3. Zivin JA. Approach to cerebrovascular disease. In: Goldman L, Ausiello D, editors. *Cecil Textbook of Medicine*. 22nd international ed. Saunders; 2004.
4. Zivin JA. Ischaemic cerebrovascular disease. In: Goldman L, Ausiello D, editors. *Cecil Textbook of Medicine*. 22nd international ed. Saunders; 2004.
5. Bak S, Gaist D, Sindrup SH, *et al*. Genetic liability in stroke: a long-term follow-up study of Danishtwins. *Stroke*. 2002; **33**: 769–74.
6. Liao D, Myers R, Hunt S, *et al*. Familial history of stroke and stroke risk: the Family Heart Study. *Stroke*. 1997; **28**: 1908–12.
7. Jousilahti P, Rastenyte D, Tuomilehto J, *et al*. Parental history of cardiovascular disease and risk of stroke: a prospective follow-up of 14 371 middle-aged men and women in Finland. *Stroke*. 1997; **28**: 1361–6.
8. Ikram MA, Seshadri S, Bis JC, *et al*. Genomewide association studies of stroke. *N Engl J Med*. 2009; **360**(17): 1718–28.

CHAPTER 3

Brain regions, lesions, and stroke syndromes

INTRODUCTION

Having reviewed the basics, we will now consider the most commonly encountered stroke syndromes. The account given herein is not meant to be exhaustive but will provide a good basic grounding in neuroanatomy and the clinical manifestations of the numerous stroke syndromes.

BRAIN REGIONS

Overview

The central nervous system consists of the brain and spinal cord. From a developmental perspective, the brain consists of three parts:

- the *forebrain*, which is made of the *cerebrum* (with its two hemispheres, each containing a cavity, the lateral ventricle) and the deeper *diencephalon* (whose main components are the thalamus, hypothalamus, and the third ventricle),
- the *midbrain* contains the aqueduct and connects the forebrain with the third portion,
- the *hindbrain*, which is made of the pons, medulla oblongata, and cerebellum (with its fourth ventricle). The midbrain, pons, and medulla oblongata form the *brainstem*.

FUNCTIONAL ANATOMY

The cerebrum

The cerebrum of the forebrain is where the apparatus of higher function resides. The surface of each hemisphere is covered with a cortex (Latin for shell or the outermost layer in anatomy) of grey matter that contains neuronal cell bodies. The surface of the cortex is characterised by tortuous folds, the *gyri*, which are separated by grooves known as the *sulci*. Some of these *sulci* (the central, lateral, and parieto-occipital sulci) divide the cerebral hemisphere to four lobes, named after their adjacent cranial bones: the *frontal lobe*, the *parietal lobe*, the *temporal lobe*, and the *occipital lobe* (*see* Figure 3.1 in the plate section).

Inside the cerebral hemispheres

The *amygdala* and the *basal ganglia* (comprising the *caudate* and the *lentiform* nuclei, the latter made up of the large lateral *putamen* and medial *globus pallidus*) lie deep within the hemispheres. The function of the amygdala will be reviewed with the limbic system as part of the temporal lobe.

Also deep in the cerebrum is the white matter of each cerebral hemisphere, which houses myelinated (and thus white) axons of three kinds: (1) axons interconnecting the two cerebral hemispheres (commissural fibres, cf. corpus callosum); (2) axons linking different parts of the same hemisphere (association fibres); and (3) axons interconnecting cortical grey matter with subcortical nuclei and the brainstem and spinal cord (projection fibres). Projection fibres consist of afferent and efferent fibres conveying impulses to the cortex and away from it. These project radially from the cortex as the *corona radiata*, which becomes concentrated in a band of white matter known as the *internal capsule*. This lies within the concavity of the caudate nucleus of particular interest to stroke, as it hosts a number of interlinking motor fibre collections.

The lobes

Each of the four lobes of each hemisphere undertakes different functions, and a reminder of these functions is worthwhile. In general terms, the dominant hemisphere is the left in right-handed people and controls speech; the non-dominant hemisphere provides more spatial awareness.

The **frontal lobe** contains centres for motor control of the opposite side of the body, insight and control of emotions, and output of speech in the dominant hemisphere. The *precentral gyrus* (*see* Figure 3.2 in the plate section) lies in front of the central sulcus (the boundary of the frontal lobe) and contains the *primary motor cortical area*, which exerts control over fine voluntary movements on the contralateral side in a somatotopic fashion as depicted by the motor homunculus (*see* Figure 3.3 in the plate section). A stroke lesion here would lead to contralateral weakness at the relevant site. The *premotor cortex*, just anteriorly to the primary motor cortex, plays a role in controlling functionally related groups of muscles. Further anteriorly lies the *frontal eye field*, responsible for voluntary conjugate deviation of the eyes; impairment of this very lesion will result in deviation of the eyes toward the side of the lesion. The *motor speech area of Broca* is in the vicinity of the lateral sulcus of the dominant hemisphere (usually left); a lesion herein would produce expressive dysphasia. The *prefrontal cortex* has important intellectual and behavioural functions, including the judging, predicting, planning, and evaluating faculties. Naturally, this convoluted role is facilitated by a rich network of interconnections between the prefrontal cortex and other brain regions. Lesions in this area can have a profound impact on aspects of human behaviour. On the inferior aspect of the frontal lobe, within its orbital surface, lies the *gyrus rectus* with the olfactory bulb, responsible for the sense of smell.

The **parietal lobe** lies just posterior to the central sulcus and above the lateral sulcus, thus behind the frontal lobe (*see* Figure 3.2). It is generally responsible for sensation in the opposite side of the body and appreciation of space, especially in the non-dominant (usually right) hemisphere. A central sulcus divides the parietal lobe into superior and inferior parietal lobules. The *postcentral gyrus* lies in the most anterior part of the parietal lobe, just behind the *central sulcus*. The *primary somatosensory cortex* resides on the surface of the postcentral gyrus. Neurons relaying information from peripheral receptors (fine and crude touch, pressure and proprioception, and pain and temperature) via the thalamus terminate in the contralateral primary somatosensory cortex. Each body part is represented in a somatotopic fashion (as depicted by the sensory homunculus; *see* Figure 3.4 in the plate section). The extent of the cortical representation is proportional to the richness of the sensory innervation that the corresponding body part requires for accomplishing its functions. Just posterior to the primary somatosensory cortex lies the vague *parietal association cortex*. This area is key to processing sensory information and spatial awareness of the opposite body site. The *superior parietal lobule* within this region is involved in interpreting somatosensory information, while the *inferior lobule* has a role in speech (in the dominant hemisphere) while also contributing to visual and auditory interrelays. Stroke affecting this area on the dominant (left) side may cause nominal dysphasia, agraphia, alexia, and acalculia. A non-dominant hemisphere stroke may render the sufferer unable to copy and construct because of spatial disorientation by precipitating constructional dyspraxia. Contralateral inferior visual loss (inferior quadrantopia) may be a result of a lesion in this region in either left or right hemisphere due to interruption of fibres (white matter) from the superior retina carrying information from the inferior visual field (the Baum's loop).

The **temporal lobe** is anatomically below the lateral sulcus. It is itself divided by two horizontal sulci into three gyri, namely the *superior, middle*, and *inferior temporal gyri*. The temporal lobe controls, broadly speaking, memory and emotions as well as comprehension of speech in the dominant hemisphere. More specifically, the *primary auditory cortex* is found on the superior temporal gyrus and receives auditory input via the medial geniculate nucleus of the thalamus. This input is subject to partial decussation prior to arrival to the thalamus and the cochleae are therefore bilaterally represented in the cortex. As a consequence, a lesion on one side does not cause deafness but partial hearing impairment. Surrounding the primary auditory cortex is the *auditory association area*. The latter contains the region known as Wernicke's area in the dominant hemisphere, which plays a crucial role in the appreciation of speech. When stroke affects this region, Wernicke's (receptive or sensory) aphasia results. Wernicke's encephalopathy does not infer pathology in this brain region but was first described by the same German physician Carl Wernicke. On the inferior surface of the temporal lobe lie the *occipito-temporal sulcus* laterally and the *collateral sulcus* medially. *Meyer's loop* is a bundle of optic radiation fibres carrying information from the inferior retina (i.e., the superior visual field) as it passes through the temporal lobe prior to reaching the visual cortex. A lesion here can cause contralateral superior quadrantopia. The *parahippocampal gyrus* lies medial to the collateral sulcus and deep into it hides the *hippocampus*. The latter projects into the floor of the lateral ventricle and is part of the limbic system. Its principal role is in regulating memory and emotions. This can rarely be involved by acute stroke (posterior cerebral artery) and may lead to complex memory deficits. The *amygdala* is found close to the anterior end of the hippocampus and is also part of the limbic system while it also receives input from the olfactory tract. Intriguing neurobehavioural constellations of symptoms may result from damage in the amygdala, which is only rarely seen in acute stroke[1] but has been reported with temporal lobe infarction (cf. Klüver-Bucy syndrome, presenting with visual agnosia, hypersexuality, placidity, hyperorality, and hypermetamorphosis).

The **occipital lobe** is found below and behind the parieto-occipital sulcus and is mostly involved in the appreciation of vision.[2] On the medial surface of the occipital lobe is the posterior part of the calcarine sulcus, and the lips of the sulcus house the *primary visual cortex*. The left visual cortex receives input from the left half of each retina, and thus the right visual field. The right visual cortex processes visual information from the right half of each retina and thus the left visual field. The precise representation is such that the upper half of the visual cortex receives from the upper half of the retina (i.e., the lower visual hemifield) with the lower half receiving input from the lower half. In other words, upper and lower visual fields are represented in a reversed order in the cortex. The posterior part of the visual cortex receives input from the macula in a fashion similar to the visual hemifields described above. Visual information is relayed via the optic radiation and the lateral geniculate nucleus of the thalamus, and blindness can be a result of interruption at any point of this anatomically sophisticated relay (*see* Figure 3.5). Occipital lobe stroke will cause contralateral homonymous hemianopia with the precise defect depending on the region of the visual cortex affected. The adjacent cortex of the occipital lobe forms the *visual association area* and this region is responsible for interpreting visual images. Lesions here would impair one's ability to recognize images and lead to visual agnosia. Occipital stroke patients with the intriguing but rare Anton-Babinski syndrome are found to be objectively blind but deny visual loss and confabulate in order to support their stance.[3]

The diencephalon

Between the cerebral hemispheres and the brainstem lies the diencephalon, where additional grey matter collections (subcortical nuclei) reside: the *epithalamus,* the *thalamus,* the *subthalamus,* and the *hypothalamus.*

The thalamus is the largest diencephalic structure and its numerous nuclei receive, amend, and convey information from key afferent, somatomotor, reticular formation, and limbic system pathways. Thalamic strokes may mimic focal cortical lesions due to the populous reciprocal thalamocortical connections. Loss of sensation in the contralateral face and limbs would be a typical thalamic deficit, often accompanied with the distressing thalamic pain experienced over the affected (anaesthetic) body areas.

The brainstem

The brainstem consists of the medulla oblongata, pons, and midbrain and links the brain and spinal cord bidirectionally, via ascending and descending tracts of white matter. The cardiovascular and respiratory centres and the cranial nerves also arise in the brainstem. There are further important agregates of grey matter known as the *colliculi,* the red, olivary, and pontine nuclei and the *reticular formation.* The latter is a diffuse system of cells and fibres that hosts the crucially important vital centres.

Within the brainstem, the pons is the portion between the midbrain and the medulla, while the medulla sits on top of the spinal cord and extends through the foramen magnum to the level of the atlas. Midbrain, pons, and medulla are linked with the cerebellum via the *superior, middle,* and *inferior cerebellar peduncles.* The top part of the medulla is bulged to a convexity on each side due to the concentrated corticospinal fibres contained within it: this structure is known as the *pyramid.* Pyramidal is the alternative name for the corticospinal tracts of fibres, the majority of which decussate at the level of the medulla prior to terminating in the grey matter of the spinal cord.

The cerebellum

The last (but not the least important) part of the hindbrain is the *cerebellum,* which sits comfortably in the posterior cranial fossa. The cerebellum is formed by the two hemispheres joined by the worm-like structure known as *cerebellar vermis.* The cerebellum also consists of an outer layer of grey matter (*cerebellar cortex*) and inner white matter. Within the deeper white matter are four pairs of nuclei that interconnect with the cerebellar cortex and with certain cell body aggregates of the brainstem and thalamus. From a functional standpoint, the cerebellum is responsible for the maintenance of equilibrium and posture and skeletal muscle tone as well as coordination of movement, all at a subconscious level. A stroke in the cerebellum will cause a lack of coordination in upper and lower limbs manifesting as hypotonia or intention tremor, dysdiadochokinesis, and an ataxic, wide-based gait. When the lesion is unilateral, the deficit is likewise. When the median *cerebellar vermis* is involved, a vertiginous labyrinthine syndrome may result that closely mimics a peripheral vestibulopathy. A cerebellar stroke can also impair eye movement by affecting the coordinated function of extraocular musculature, thereby leading to nystagmus with the fast component pointing toward the side of the lesion. Dysarthria may ensue but is not sign specific to stroke, as it is commonly seen with bilateral cerebellar involvement, as in alcohol intoxication, hypothyroidism, and multiple sclerosis.

The spinal cord

The spinal cord, which is buried protected within the vertebral column, is in continuity with the brain via the medulla, the lowest portion of the brainstem. The topographical anatomy of the spinal cord is as complex as the numerous ascending and descending tracts that it relays (*see* Figures 3.2 and 3.3) but a basic understanding is crucial to appreciating how the neural circuitry is interlinked.

Its central H-shaped core of grey matter (cell bodies) can be divided into *posterior (dorsal)*, *lateral*, and *anterior (ventral) horns*. The tip of the posterior horn is also known as *substantia gelatinosa*, important for transmission of nociceptive impulses. The origin of the contralateral *spinothalamic* tract (*nucleus proprius*) and *Clarke's column* (mediating tactile, pressure, and impulses from muscle fibres) are also located in the posterior horn. The preganglionic sympathetic neuron cell bodies (thoracolumbar) are found in the lateral horn of the grey matter horn. There is a small group of preganglionic cell bodies in the lateral horn of the sacral segments (S2–S4), which are the origin of the pelvic splanchnic nerves. Lastly, the ventral (anterior) is home to alpha and gamma motor neurones, also known as lower motor neurons. The more medial anterior horn cells innervate the musculature of the trunk while the more lateral cells of that group supply the limb muscles.

The mantle of white matter surrounding the H-shaped grey matter core contains fibres making ascending tracts carrying information via a chain of three neurons (from peripheral receptor to brain). The most important ascending tracts can be seen as two distinct groups: the *lateral and anterior white columns* and the *posterior (dorsal) white columns*. The former mediate pain (nociception) and temperature, crude touch (pressure), itch, tickle, sexual orgasm, as well as muscular coordination via interconnections with the cerebellum. The latter are made of the gracile and cuneate tracts and more concerned with discriminative (light) touch, vibration, and proprioception sense as well as the sense of fullness of bladder and rectum. The spinocerebellar tracts (ventral and dorsal) carry unconscious proprioceptive signals from spinal cord to cerebellum.

An important group of descending fibres is the lower *corticospinal tract*, which is made of the decussated medullary motor fibres. Because of that decussation, each side of the body is essentially controlled by the contralateral hemisphere. The lateral and medial reticulospinal tracts convey information from the medullary and pontine reticular formation, respectively. The lateral vestibulospinal tract (depicted in Figure 3.3) originates from the vestibular nucleus of the medulla and terminates in truncal and limb musculature.

The exact ensuing clinical syndrome depends on the location of the spinal cord lesion and results from destruction at segmental level on a par with the interruption of the ascending and descending tracts, whether sensory or motor. An *upper cervical cord lesion* would therefore lead to spastic tetraparesis with exaggerated reflexes and positive Babinski sign (upper motor neuron deficit). Incontinence, sensory loss, and sensory ataxia below the level of the lesion will also ensue. With a *lower cervical cord lesion*, parts of the upper limbs will be afflicted in a lower motor neuron pattern, with weakness, muscle wasting, fasciculation, and reduced reflexes. The lower limbs will be affected in an upper motor neuron (UMN) pattern, as described above. The clinical manifestations of thoracic and lumbar lesions will obey a similar pattern. A hemilesion is a somewhat interesting entity, historically known as Brown-Sequard syndrome, manifesting with ipsilateral loss of proprioception and UMN signs associated with contralateral loss of pain and temperature.

Neurovasculature

The brain is provided with arterial blood by two pairs of vessels: the internal carotid arteries and the vertebral arteries. The right and left internal carotid arteries and their branching vessels make the anterior circulation. The vertebral arteries and their branches form the posterior circulation. Anterior and posterior circulations are adjoined by means of the posterior communicating arteries to form the Circle of Willis.[2]

Anterior circulation

The internal carotid arteries arise from each of the common carotid arteries and follow a rather adventurous course, full of bends and turns, as they enter the cranial cavity through the carotid canal. That tortuous path is responsible for the name of part of the artery, the carotid siphon. Each internal carotid artery subsequently passes through the cavernous sinus and the hypophyseal arteries, supplying the neurohypophysis, come off from the intracavernous portion of the internal carotid. As the latter emerges from the roof of the cavernous sinus, it gives off the preterminal ophthalmic artery. The ophthalmic artery passes into the orbit through the optic foramen to supply the various orbital structures, as well as the dorsum of the nose, the frontal and ethmoidal sinuses, and the frontal part of the scalp. The parent internal carotid artery subsequently turns upward and gives rise to the middle and anterior cerebral arteries, terminal arteries supplying the cerebral cortex.

At the same level, it also gives rise to the preterminal anterior choroidal and the posterior communicating arteries. The former rarely arises from the middle cerebral artery and is distributed to the optic tract and radiation, the lateral geniculate body, the choroid plexus of the lateral ventricle, some basal ganglia, parts of the limbic system, and the posterior limb of the internal capsule.

The middle cerebral artery (MCA) is the largest of the three cerebral vessels and, being an almost direct continuation of the internal carotid, is very prone to embolism. It passes into the lateral sulcus to supply the insula and the auditory cortex prior to reaching and supplying the lateral hemisphere (frontal, parietal, and temporal lobes) almost in its entirety. In functional terms, the middle cerebral artery supplies the primary motor and sensory cortices for the contralateral body side except for the perineum, leg, and foot. The latter three bodies are supplied by the anterior cerebral artery. Striate branches (also known as perforating, lenticulostriate, thalamostriate, and thalamolenticular) arising from the origin of the MCA reach the internal capsule, the thalamus, and basal ganglia. The Broca's and Wernicke's areas (in the dominant hemisphere) are important brain regions also supplied by the middle cerebral artery. One approach to further describing MCA anatomy is in a segmental manner, whereby brain landmarks are used to divide the vessel in segments (M1, M2, M3, and M4). In the slightly more practical functional branching approach, the superior and inferior branches of the middle cerebral artery are examined separately on the basis that they supply functionally distinct brain regions. The *superior division* of the MCA supplies the frontal and superior parietal lobes, whereas the *inferior division* supplies inferior parietal and temporal lobes.

The anterior cerebral artery (ACA) arises as the medial branch of the bifurcation of the internal carotid (ICA) at the level of the anterior clinoid process. The anterior cerebral artery passes above the optic nerve and into the great longitudinal fissure between the frontal lobes. It is joined to its mirror vessel from the contralateral hemicranium by the short anterior communicating artery. The ACA supplies the whole of the medial surface of each hemisphere above the corpus callosum and extending back up to the parieto-occipital sulcus (below and behind which lies the occipital lobe). It thus supplies the medial surface of the frontal and parietal lobes and its territory includes the motor and sensory cortices for the contralateral perineum, leg, and foot as well as micturition and defaecation.

Posterior circulation

The vertebral arteries arise from the subclavian arteries and course through the foramen magnum into the cranium prior to converging at the junction between medulla and pons to form the basilar artery. Each vertebral artery gives rises to the *anterior* and *posterior spinal arteries*, supplying the medulla and spinal cord, and the renowned *posterior inferior cerebellar artery*, supplying the inferior part of the cerebellum.

The midline basilar artery runs up in front of the pons to give off the small pontine branches, which supply, as their name betrays, the pons. The *anterior inferior cerebellar artery* and the *labyrinthine artery* are also branches of the basilar artery and supply anterior and inferior cerebellum and inner ear, respectively. The basilar artery ascends up and ends at the upper end of the pons by dividing into the *superior cerebellar branches* just before giving rise to the *posterior cerebral arteries*. The former supplies the remaining superior part of the cerebellum, as well as the mesencephalon and upper pons. The posterior cerebral artery supplies the visual cortex of the occipital lobe (but the macula can be MCA-supplied). The inferomedial portion of the temporal lobe, posterior and inferior parts of parietal, and the lateral thalamus (via the thalamogeniculate branch) are also supplied by the PCA. It should be noted that the posterior cerebral artery may receive some of its blood from the internal carotid and not the basilar, the basilar artery being a later embryological development. A number of perforating arteries arising from the posterior cerebral or the posterior communicating arteries (*see* below) supply the anterior part of the midbrain and aspects of subthalamus and hypothalamus. In summary, the *posterior cerebral arteries* are crucial to the occipital lobes, midbrain, thalamus, and parts of the temporal and parietal lobes.

The vertebrobasilar system communicates with the anterior circulation with the aid of the two thin *posterior communicating arteries*, thus forming the anastomosis known as *circulus arteriosus* or *Circle of Willis*, so named after the English physician Thomas Willis. This vascular circle surrounds the floor of the hypothalamus, the optic chiasma, and the midbrain and provides, when the communicating vessels are patent and fully functional, opportunity for compensatory flow in case of vascular compromise.

ISCHAEMIC SYNDROMES

Carotid artery lesions

Common and internal carotid lesions may result in stroke by embolisation and subsequent occlusion of the intracranial vessels. Young people with isolated carotid artery occlusive disease may be completely asymptomatic but unilateral blindness is characteristic of ICA occlusion. This results from involvement of the retinal artery, which is a branch of the ophthalmic artery. However, in most cases, carotid artery territory stroke will cause clinical features such as hemiparesis or dysphasia (when the dominant hemisphere is affected) and other features, depending on the vessel afflicted.

An extremely rare entity, first described by Miller Fisher in 1962, is the limb-shaking syndrome associated with carotid stenosis.[5] Despite its rare occurrence, it is important to recognise as it may easily be misdiagnosed as focal seizure but is a feature of high vascular risk.

The MCA syndromes

The middle cerebral artery has been described as the most complex of the major cerebral arteries and its branches are the most commonly affected by cerebral infarction. Occlusion of the middle cerebral artery or any of its 'daughter' vessels is most commonly due to an embolic event rather than intrinsic vascular pathology.[6]

Complete MCA occlusion will commonly be dramatic with variable clinical signs, depending on the availability of collateral cortical supply. Resulting clinical manifestations comprise:

- **contralateral hemiplegia**
- **hemianaesthesia**
- **contralateral homonymous hemianopia**
- **gaze preference to the ipsilateral side** (i.e., looking toward the side of the damage)
- **conjugate ocular deviation**
- **dysarthria** (due to facial weakness)
- **global dysphasia** (dominant hemisphere)
- **anosognosia** (non-dominant hemisphere)
- **contralateral hemispatial neglect** (non-dominant hemisphere).

The term 'malignant MCA syndrome' denotes rapid deterioration secondary to cerebral oedema accompanying a large MCA infarct. Brainstem compression may culminate even in death and the caring physician should be alarmed by any early signs of neurological decline, even as subtle as cephalgia and vomiting.[7] There is evidence to suggest that, in selected cases, surgical decompression (by craniotomy) of patients with large, swollen MCA infarcts improves survival.

When the superior or inferior divisions of the MCA are involved in isolation, an incomplete syndrome will ensue: e.g., occlusion of superior branches leads to Broca's dysphasia (if dominant) and contralateral lower face and arm weakness or neglect (if non-dominant); inferior branch lesions on the other hand may cause Wernicke's dysphasia (if dominant) or constructional apraxia (if non-dominant), contra-lateral visual field defects with hemi-neglect, aprosody (loss of normal pitch and rhythm in speech), and anosognosia (denial of a neurological deficit such as hemiparesis).

Anterior cerebral artery syndrome

Occlusion of this artery (often embolic) is much less common than MCA territory infarction. As discussed earlier, this vessel supplies the medial surface of the frontal and parietal lobes and its territory includes the motor and sensory cortices for the contralateral perineum, leg, and foot as well as micturition and defaecation. Characteristic neurological manifestations that typically result from ACA infarction therefore comprise:

- **motor deficits** (paralysis of the contralateral leg, involuntary resistance to passive movement of affected limb)

- **sphincter dysfunction** (urinary incontinence)
- **language disorders** (perseveration)
- **pathological grasp phenomena**
- **alien limb syndrome, amnesia**
- (and more rarely) **sensory deficits, akinetic mutism, abulia,** and **other psychomotor disorders.**

Anterior choroidal artery syndrome

This rare syndrome was originally described by Foix in 1925.[8] When complete, it classically manifests with the triad of:
- **hemiplegia,**
- **hemisensory loss,** and
- **homonymous hemianopia,** all contralateral to the lesion.

Infarction typically involves the posterior limb of the internal capsule, the lateral geniculate body, and the globus pallidus. Dominant hemisphere lesions may result to speech disorders, and non-dominant deficits will be associated with spatial neglect in the less complete forms of the lesion.[9]

Posterior cerebral artery syndrome

The most frequent clinical finding is contralateral **hemianopia** with relative macular sparing. If the parietal lobe is involved, the resultant anosagnosia implies that the patient may not be aware of the visual deficit. Thalamic involvement (by infarction of the thalamogeniculate branch) may lead to contralateral **hemisensory** signs, the second most common constellation of clinical findings in PCA territory infarction. These can be slight but usually include paraesthesia and numbness. Dominant (left) hemisphere lesions affecting the parieto-occipital region can also cause **reading abnormalities (alexia without agraphia).** **Visual agnosia** may also complicate left-sided PCA infarction and may result in inability to name objects but the object can be readily identified via tactile and auditory recognition. **Persistent amnesia** and inability to form new memories may also result from left medial temporal lobe involvement. Contralateral visual **neglect** can also occur, particularly with right-sided infarction, while hemi-motor deficits are generally rare. Bilateral PCA territory infarction could render the patient **cortically blind,** nonetheless adamant that they can see (**Anton's syndrome**). Disorientation, hyperactivity, and even hypotension may also accompany bilateral posterior cerebral artery injury.[10]

Cerebellar syndromes

Posterior circulation ischaemia must be recognised early as its consequences can be particularly serious and readily available non-contrast CT imaging provides poor resolution of some cerebellar and brainstem lesions. Clinical signs depend of the branch of the cerebellar vasculature involved and the clinical picture is frequently perplexed by involvement of additional territories. The main cerebellar stroke syndromes are categorised on the basis of the vascular territory involved by the infarct, as follows.

- **Superior cerebellar artery (rarely affected in isolation).** May involve the superior surface of cerebellum, thalamic and subthalamic regions, occipital and temporal lobes, and upper pons. Classically manifests with dysarthria, headache, dizziness, vomiting, and ataxia; also ipsilateral limb dysmetria and Horner's; contralateral loss of pain and temperature sensation; contralateral CN IV palsy.
- **Anterior inferior cerebellar artery (rarely affected in isolation).** May affect the lateral aspect of lower pons. Classically manifests with dysarthria, headache, dizziness, vomiting, and ataxia; also ipsilateral limb dysmetria and Horner's; contralateral loss of pain and temperature sensation; ipsilateral CN V, VII, and VIII palsies.
- **Posterior inferior cerebellar artery.** Affects dorsal lateral medullary area. Classically manifests with dysarthria, headache, dizziness, vomiting, and ataxia.

Brainstem syndromes

Extensive brainstem infarction is bound to be associated with extensive neurology, with the precise clinical picture depending on the precise anatomical damage incurred.[18] Important brainstem stroke syndromes are summarised below.

- **Locked-in syndrome.** Produced by occlusion of proximal and middle segments of the important basilar artery, supplying the *basis pontis*. Classically manifests as quadriplegia with spared awareness (due to upper pons sparing); also lower cranial nerve deficits.
- **Top of the basilar syndrome.** Due to distal basilar artery segment occlusion producing rostral midbrain and thalamus infarction. Oculomotor signs may include poorly reactive pupils and vertical gaze deficits. May be accompanied by impaired consciousness, somnolence, vivid hallucinations, amnesia, and agitation.[19]
- **Weber's syndrome.** Named after the German-born Sir Weber; with an infarct afflicting lateral and paramedian midbrain, manifests with ipsilateral CN III palsy and contralateral hemiplegia.
- **Lateral medullary syndrome** (German internist and neurologist **Wallenberg's syndrome**). Ataxia, vertigo, nystagmus; nausea and vomiting; ipsilateral Horner's syndrome; ipsilateral facial and body sensory loss; swallowing and speaking difficulties. Due to lateral medullary infarction.
- **Benedict's syndrome.** Named after Hungarian-Austrian neurologist Moritz Benedikt; ipsilateral CN III palsy and involuntary abnormal movements affecting lower limbs are the classic manifestations due to paramedian upper midbrain and red nucleus infarction.
- **Claude's syndrome.** Named after French psychiatrist and neurologist Henri Claude; is produced by paramedian upper midbrain and cerebro-thalamic connection infarction; manifests with ipsilateral CN III palsy and contralateral cerebellar signs.

Lacunar syndromes

Lacunar infarcts are small deep infarcts that occur in the territory of the various deep penetrating arteries. Such affected vessels are the lenticulostriate, the anterior striate and Heubner arteries of the MCA, the thalamoperforators of the PCA, and deep perforators of the basilar artery. Infarcts in these vessels can produce a variety of features, but the classic syndromes are as follows.

1 **Pure motor stroke**: the commonest in clinical practice, often involving internal capsule and basis pontis; the signs (whether on face or limbs) are accurately summarised by the name of this syndrome.
2 **Pure sensory stroke**: not as common as its motor counterpart and often due to small deep infarcts often affecting the thalamus by involving the corresponding perforators.
3 **Sensorimotor stroke**: reasonably common and due to small deep infarct involving internal capsule, thalamocortical pathways, or corona radiata.
4 **Dysarthria-clumsy hand syndrome**: originally described as a syndrome involving dysarthria and clumsiness of one hand, due to a pontine lacune.
5 **Ataxic hemiparesis**: a syndrome of unilateral weakness and ataxia, due to small deep infarcts typically in the vicinity of the internal capsule, thalamus, corona radiate, and less commonly the lentiform nucleus.[11]

HAEMORRHAGIC STROKES

These are less common than their ischaemic counterparts[12] but their accompanying deficits are often more severe and associated with high mortality.[13] Modern imaging modalities have enabled the accurate and early recognition of intracranial haemorrhage.[14] Clinical features again depend on the area of brain involved and are often associated with general features such as headache, vomiting, and rapid or progressive onset. While these suggest haemorrhage rather than infarction, it remains impossible to identify haemorrhage with certainty on purely clinical grounds.

- **Putaminal haemorrhage** typically features contralateral flaccid hemiparesis, contralateral hemisensory loss, contralateral conjugate gaze paresis, homonymous hemianopia, dysphasia, and unilateral spatial neglect. The deficits typically progress and are frequently accompanied by headache and vomiting. Haemorrhage originates from the lenticulostriate arteries supplying the putamen, with their lateral branches being the most common culprit.[15]
- **Thalamic haemorrhage** may manifest with contralateral hemiparesis, contralateral sensory loss, homonymous hemianopia, vertical gaze abnormalities, miosis, aphasia, and confusion. Neuropsychiatric disturbances, impaired consciousness, and minimal motor or sensory deficits may be seen in restricted bleeds. The origin of the haemorrhage may be from any of the four arterial pedicles supplying the thalamus, which in turn receive their blood supply from the basilar, the posterior communicating, and the proximal portions of the posterior cerebral arteries.[16]

- **Lobar haemorrhage** may cause contralateral hemiparesis (especially with frontal bleeds) or sensory loss (severe in parietal haematomas), contralateral conjugate gaze paresis (with frontal and temporal haemorrhage), homonymous hemianopia (with occipital, parietal, and temporal haemorrhage), dysphasia (in frontal, temporal, and parieral haemorrhage), neglect (with temporal and parietal damage), abulia (with frontal bleeds), or apraxia (common with parietal haematomas). Clinical signs and symptoms will vary and depend on the anatomical regions involved.[17]
- **Brainstem haemorrhage** can have catastrophic clinical sequelae in a manner similar to infarction. Quadriparesis, decreased level of consciousness, gaze paresis, miosis, and facial weakness are some of the clinical features accompanying haemorrhagic damage in this critical area.[18]
- **Cerebellar haemorrhage** may manifest with acute posterior headache and ataxia, drowsiness, vertigo, vomiting, dysarthria, nystagmus, or even coma. The perforating branches of the superior cerebellar artery are fragile and commonly complicated by haemorrhage. Appropriate neuroimaging is essential to diagnosis as cerebellar infarction may present with a clinically identical pattern.

REFERENCES

1. Chou CL, Lin YJ, Sheu YL, *et al*. Persistent Kuver-Bucy syndrome after temporal lobe infarction. *Acta Neurol Taiwan*. 2008; **17**(3): 199–202.
2. Crossman AR, Neary D. *Neuroanatomy: an illustrated colour text*. 2nd ed. Churchill Livingstone; 1995.
3. Maddula M, Lutton S, Keegan B. Anton's syndrome due to cerebrovascular disease: a case report. *J Med Case Reports*. 2009; **3**: 9028.
4. Fuller G, Manford M. *Neurology: an illustrated colour text*. Churchill Livingstone; 2006.
5. Kowacz PA, Troiano AR, Mendonca CT, *et al*. Carotid transient ischemic attacks presenting as limb-shaking syndrome. *Arq Neuropsiquiatr*. 2004; **62**(2–A): 339–41.
6. Neau J-P, Bogousslavsky J. Superficial middle cerebral artery syndromes. In: Bogousslavsky J, Caplan L, editors. *Stroke Syndromes*. 2nd ed. Cambridge University Press; 2001.
7. Treadwell SD, Thanvi B. Malignant middle cerebral artery (MCA) infarction: pathophysiology, diagnosis and management. *Postgrad Med J*. 2010; **86**(1014): 235–42.
8. Foix CH, Chaveny JA, Hillemand P, *et al*. Obliteration de l'artere Choroldienne anterieure. Ramollissement de son territoire cerebral. Hemiplegie, hemianesthesie, Hemianopsie. *Bulletin de la Societi d'Ophtalmologie de Parb*. 1925; 37: 221–3.
9. Decroix JP, Graveleau PH, Masson M, *et al*. Infarction in the territory of the anterior choroidal artery. *Brain*. 1986; **109**(6): 1071–85.
10. Chaves CJ, Caplan LR. Posterior cerebral artery. In: Bogousslavsky J, Caplan L, editors. *Stroke Syndromes*. 2nd ed. Cambridge University Press; 2001.
11. Bamford JM. Classical lacunar syndromes. In: Bogousslavsky J, Caplan L, editors. *Stroke Syndromes*. 2nd ed. Cambridge University Press; 2001.
12. Warlow C, Dennis M, van Gijn J, *et al*. *Stroke: a practical guide to management*. 2nd ed. Blackwell Sciences Limited; 2001.

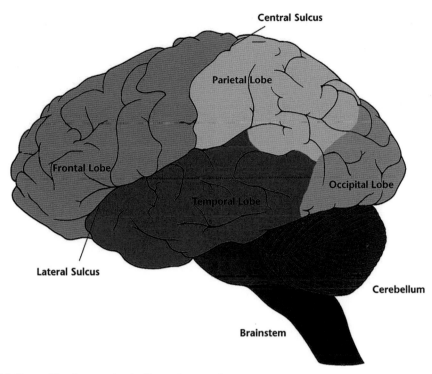

FIGURE 3.1 The human brain (lateral aspect)

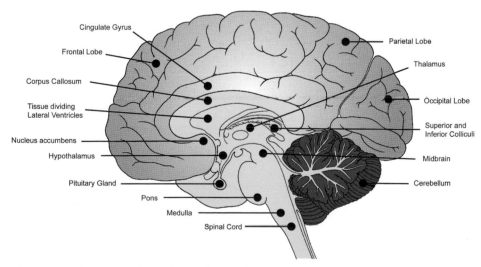

FIGURE 3.2 The human brain (medial aspect)

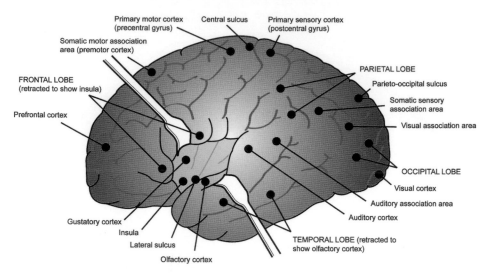

FIGURE 3.3 Sulci and gyri and lobes

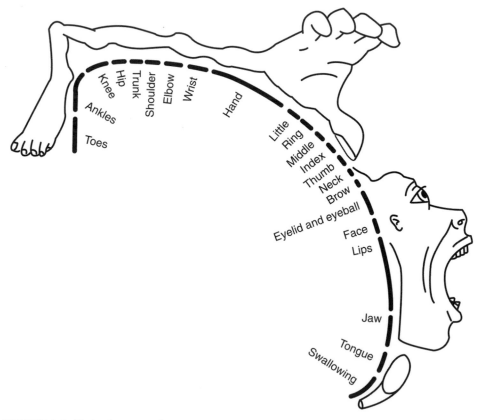

FIGURE 3.4 Motor homunculus

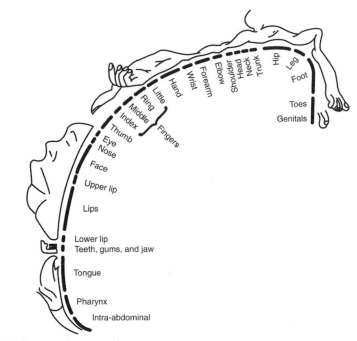

FIGURE 3.5 Sensory homunculus

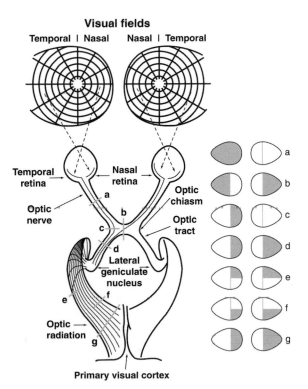

FIGURE 3.6 Visual pathways from eye to brain

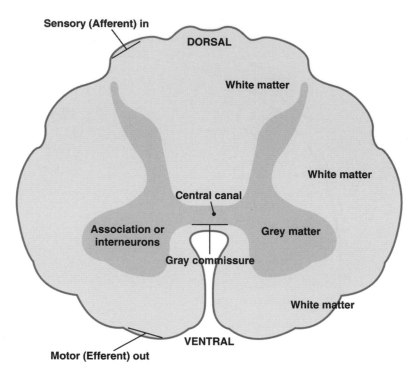

FIGURE 3.7 The internal structure of the spinal cord

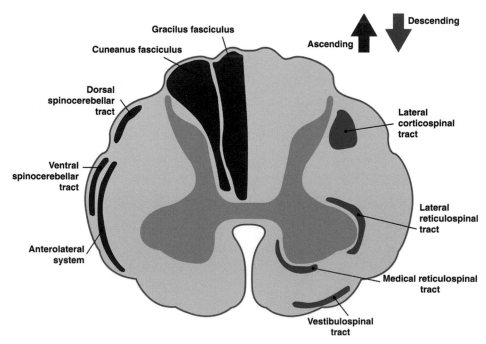

FIGURE 3.8 Ascending and descending spinal cord tracts

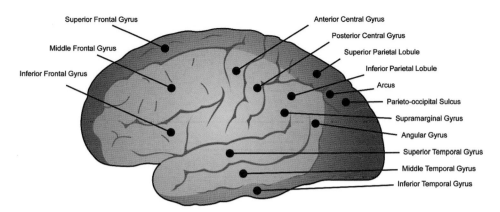

FIGURE 3.9 Lateral aspect of cerebral hemisphere illustrating areas supplied by arteries (middle cerebral artery [MCA] territory shown as pink, anterior cerebral artery [ACA] as blue, and posterior cerebral artery [PCA] as yellow)

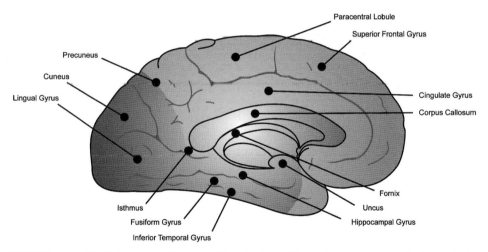

FIGURE 3.10 Medial aspect of cerebral hemisphere illustrating areas supplied by arteries (MCA territory shown as pink, ACA as blue, and PCA as yellow)

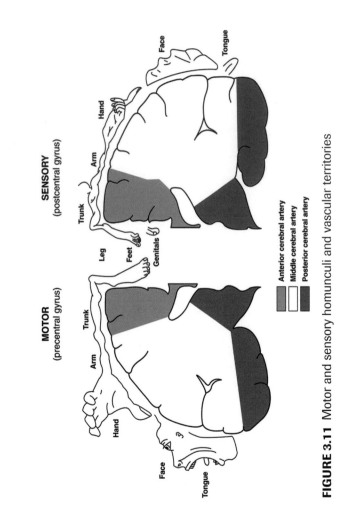

FIGURE 3.11 Motor and sensory homunculi and vascular territories

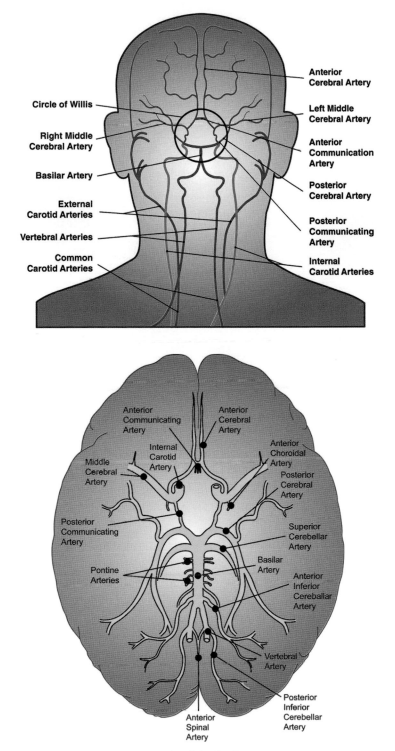

FIGURES 3.12 AND 3.13 Arterial supply of the brain

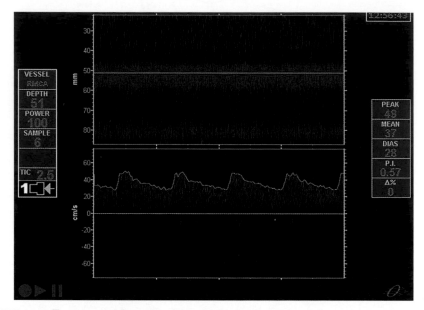

FIGURE 10.7 Transcranial Doppler ultrasound trace from the right middle cerebral artery. The yellow line in the top panel indicates the depth at which the lower spectral trace is obtained. The flow velocity at this depth is shown in the far right panel and is toward the lower limit of normal. The thick red trace in the top panel (from 46 to 58 mm) represents a 12 mm segment of the middle cerebral artery

13. Demaerschalk BM, Aguilar MI. Treatment of acute intracerebral hemorrhage. *Curr Treat Options Neurol*. 2008; **10**(6): 455–67.

14. Fisher M. Primary intracerebral and subarachnoid hemorrhage. An approach to diagnosis and therapy. *Arq Neuropsiquiatr*. 1991; **49**(3): 233–42.

15. Minematsu K, Yamaguchi T. Putaminal haemorrhages. In: Bogousslavsky J, Caplan L, editors. *Stroke Syndromes*. 2nd ed. Cambridge University Press; 2001.

16. Barth A, Bogousslavsky J, Caplan IR. Thalamic infarcts and haemorrhages. In: Bogousslavsky J, Caplan L, editors. *Stroke Syndromes*. 2nd ed. Cambridge University Press; 2001.

17. Kase C. Lobar haemorrhages. In: Bogousslavsky J, Caplan L, editors. *Stroke Syndromes*. 2nd ed. Cambridge University Press; 2001.

18. Tettenborn BE. Extended infarcts in the posterior circulation (brainstem/cerebellum). In: Bogousslavsky J, Caplan L, editors. *Stroke Syndromes*. 2nd ed. Cambridge University Press; 2001.

19. Caplan LR. 'Top of the basilar' syndrome. *Neurology*. 1980; **30**(1): 72–9.

FURTHER READING

• Moore KL, Dalley AF, Agur AMR. *Clinically Oriented Anatomy*. 6th revised international ed. Lippincott Williams and Wilkins; 2009.

• Sinnatamby CS. *Last's Anatomy: regional and applied*. 10th ed. Churchill Livingstone; 1999.

• Whitaker RH, Borley NR. *Instant Anatomy*. 4th ed. Wiley-Blackwell; 2010.

• Drake R, Vogl AW, Mitchell AWM. *Gray's Anatomy for Students*. 2nd ed. Churchill Livingstone; 2009.

CHAPTER 4

Classification

OUTLINE

Stroke is a heterogeneous disease entity underlined by numerous but frequently overlapping pathophysiological processes. Stroke classification can thus be just as heterogeneous. There are a number of ways to classify stroke, but only the two main and most widely known classification systems will be discussed. Classification systems based on features such as stroke duration and evolution are not widely employed and no reference to them is made herein.[1]

PATHOPHYSIOLOGICAL CLASSIFICATION

This divides stroke into ischaemic and haemorrhagic subtypes and each of these is further subdivided as shown in Table 4.1. The subdivision of ischaemic stroke is based on the prototype classification as proposed by Kunitz, *et al.* in the Stroke Databank pilot study[2] incorporating elements from the classification proposed by Adams, *et al.* (TOAST classification).[3]

TABLE 4.1 Pathophysiological classification of stroke

Ischaemic stroke
Thrombotic (usually atherosclerotic, affecting large arteries)
Embolic
Lacunar (small vessel disease)
Other undetermined pathology
Multiple possible pathologies
Cerebral haemorrhage (non-traumatic)
Intraparenchymal haemorrhage
Subdural haemorrhage
Mixed (e.g., vascular malformations)

Thrombosis usually occurs due to underlying atherosclerosis and most frequently affects the extracerebral carotid system and the basilar artery. Embolism most commonly involves the intracerebral arteries (most frequently the middle cerebral artery distribution). Emboli can originate from cardiac mural thrombi, valvular disease, and atrial fibrillation. Fragments of thrombotic material can arise from arterial mural thrombi (most often in the carotid artery), or more rarely as paradoxical emboli. Lacunar infarcts result from occlusion of deep perforating arteries that arise from both the anterior and posterior circulations and supply the white matter of the cerebral hemispheres and brainstem.

Haemorrhage accounts for some 20% of stroke presentations with intraparenchymal haemorrhage being the most common subtype, often described as either

TABLE 4.2 Oxford or Bamford classification

Syndrome	*Features*
Total anterior circulation infarct (TACI)	All of these: • Higher dysfunction (dysphasia, visuospatial) • Homonymous hemianopia • Motor/sensory deficit

Partial anterior circulation infarct (PACI)	Any one of these:
	• Two out of three as TACI
	  1 Higher dysfunction (dysphasia, visuospatial)
	  2 Homonymous hemianopia
	  3 Motor/sensory deficit
	    > 2/3 face/arm/leg
	• Higher dysfunction alone
	• Limited motor/sensory deficit

Posterior circulation infarct (POCI)	Any of these features • Cranial nerve palsy AND contralateral motor/sensory deficit • Bilateral motor or sensory deficit • Conjugate eye movement problems • Cerebellar dysfunction WITHOUT ipsilateral long tract signs • Isolated homonymous hemianopia
Lacunar infarction (LACI)	Any one of these: • Pure motor stroke (2/3 of face/arm/leg) • Pure sensory stroke (2/3 of face/arm/leg) • Sensorimotor stroke (2/3 of face/arm/leg) • Ataxic hemiparesis Must have none of these: • New dysphasia • New visuospatial problem • Proprioceptive sensory loss only • Vertebrobasilar features

hypertensive or lobar haemorrhage. Subarachnoid haemorrhage typically follows rupture of a berry aneurysm.

CLINICAL CLASSIFICATION

Bamford, *et al.* first described the incidence and natural history of four clinically identifiable subgroups of cerebral infarction in an Oxfordshire community-based study in a landmark paper published in the *Lancet* in 1991.[4] This account is now widely adopted and utilised as the clinical classification of stroke syndromes known as the eponymous Bamford or Oxford classification.

In this system, cerebral infarction is divided into four categories: total anterior circulation infarction (TACI), partial anterior circulation infarction (PACI), lacunar infarction (LACI), and posterior circulation infarction (POCI). The basis of the Oxford classification system is the apparent pathoanatomical location of the lesion as manifested by symptoms and signs. The aetiology of the different subtypes can be overlapping, as each subtype may be due to same pathology only manifesting in distinct loci. It comes as no surprise that this classification, despite being universally employed by clinicians, is regarded as less suited for aetiological studies.

It should be noted that the same system is used to describe stroke of haemorrhagic aetiology, although this was not the subject of the original paper.

The Oxford classification remains indispensable to clinical practice because of its prognostic significance. Indeed, total anterior circulation infarcts (TACI) carry the worst prognosis in terms of death or disability. Posterior (POCI), partial (PACI), and lacunar infarcts (LACI) have a better prognosis but PACIs have a high risk of recurrent stroke within three months.

REFERENCES

1. Boon N, Colledge N, Walker B. Neurology. In: *Davidson's Principles and Practice of Medicine*. 20th international ed. Churchill Livingstone; 2006.
2. Kunitz SC, Gross CRE, Heyman A, *et al*. The pilot Stroke Data Bank: definition, design, and data. *Stroke*. 1984; **15**: 740–6.
3. Adams HP Jr, Davis PH, Leira EC, *et al*. Baseline NIH Stroke Scale score strongly predicts outcome after stroke: A report of the Trial of Org 10172 in Acute Stroke Treatment (TOAST). *Neurology*. 1999; **53**(1): 126–31.
4. Bamford J, Sandercock P, Dennis M, *et al*. Classification and natural history of clinically identifiable subtypes of cerebral infarction. *Lancet*. 1991; **337**(8756): 1521–6.

CHAPTER 5

Assessment of the stroke patient

INTRODUCTION

This chapter gives practical advice for the hospital assessment of stroke patients, both on admission and during their hospital stay. This includes clinical evaluation at the bedside, basic laboratory investigations, and non-invasive brain and vascular imaging. The purpose of assessment is to initially assess clinical state, try to determine aetiology, and guide appropriateness for acute management strategies such as thrombolytic therapy for ischaemic stroke. Stroke mimics can usually be identified at this stage, should the pre-hospital survey have missed it. Progress post admission needs to be monitored and regularly assessed and this includes further clinical assessment, more specialised neurovascular imaging, and other tests (discussed in other chapters).

PRE-HOSPITAL ASSESSMENT

Stroke assessment can be subdivided into pre-hospital and hospital assessment. A number of assessment tools have been developed in order to aid the prompt and accurate identification of stroke in the community and in primary care. Tools such as the Los Angeles Prehospital Stroke Screen (LAPSS) (*see* Table 5.1), the Cincinnati Prehospital Stroke Scale (CPSS) (*see* Table 5.2), and the Newcastle Face Arm Speech Test (FAST) (*see* Table 5.3) have been developed. Each of these has different sensitivity and specificity and their own advantages and drawbacks but all serve nearly equally well their primary aim, which is to rapidly identify stroke.

TABLE 5.1 Los Angeles Prehospital Stroke Scale (LAPSS) screening criteria1

1 Age >45

2 No history of seizures or epilepsy

3 Symptom duration <24 hrs

4 At baseline, patient is not wheelchair bound or bedridden

5 Blood glucose between 60 and 400

6 Obvious unilateral asymmetry (right versus left), i.e., facial smile/grimace; grip; arm strength

If 1–6 are yes with asymmetry on exam, then LAPSS criteria are met and stroke is assumed to have occurred.

TABLE 5.2 Cincinnati Prehospital Stroke Scale (CPSS)

Facial droop: have patient smile, show teeth
Normal if both sides of face move equally
Abnormal if one side of face does not move or does not move as well as the other

Arm drift: arms held out straight in front of body with eyes closed for 10s
Normal if both arms move equally or not at all
Abnormal if one arm unable to maintain position or drifts compared to the other

Speech: have patient repeat a phrase
Normal if patient uses correct words, no slurring
Abnormal if slurred words, inappropriate words, or unable to speak

If any of the above tests are abnormal, stroke is assumed to have occurred.

TABLE 5.3 Face Arm Speech Test (FAST)

Speech impairment: slurring or expressive difficulties

Facial palsy: asymmetry

Arm weakness: monitor arms held out for five seconds and document side of drift/weakness

Time to call 999—if any of the above features are present, stroke is assumed to have occurred.

IMMEDIATE HOSPITAL ASSESSMENT

Diagnosis

Stroke diagnosis is the composite of accurate clinical history and physical assessment, the cornerstone of which is the neurological examination. The immediate physical assessment of the stroke patient should be rapid but accurate. A rapid scheme for establishing clinical history and examination is presented in Tables 5.4 and 5.5 but a more complete approach is discussed subsequently.

TABLE 5.4 History

Headache?
Nausea?
Vomiting?

Vertigo?
Ataxia?

Visual Disturbance?
Diplopia?

Language Disorder?
Dysarthria?

Limb Weakness?
Paraesthesiae?

TABLE 5.5 Examination

GCS And Mental State

Higher Cortical Function

Cranial Nerves

Visual Fields
Fundoscopy

Upper And Lower Limbs: Tone, Power, Reflexes/Sensation/Coordination

Pulse/BP/Cardiac Murmurs/Carotid Bruits

Severity

A useful algorithm for assessing the severity of stroke patient in the immediate setting is the National Institute of Health Stroke Scale (NIHSS). This should be done as soon as stroke is diagnosed as it conveys important prognostic information and may help inform the use of treatments such as thrombolytic therapy.

It provides a rapid and reproducible means of quantifying neurological deficit and can thus be used to monitor progress over time; any increase in NIHSS score should prompt more thorough assessment for complications such as recurrent stroke or cerebral oedema. It is important to acknowledge it is not a diagnostic scale but can of course help identify those with stroke.

We do not recommend a very detailed neurological examination in the immediate setting in the thrombolysis candidate. The scale is presented in Table 5.6. To perform a NIHSS assessment, it is important to perform the examination in the presented order and to score patients as they perform, not as you believe they may on repeated assessment.

TABLE 5.6 NIH scale

Instructions	*Scale definition*
1a Level of consciousness:	**0** = Alert; keenly responsive. **1** = Not alert, but arousable by minor stimulation to obey, answer, or respond. **2** = Not alert, requires repeated stimulation to attend, or is obtunded and requires strong or painful stimulation to make movements (not stereotyped). **3** = Responds only with reflex motor or autonomic effects or totally unresponsive, flaccid, or areflexic.
1b LOC questions: Ask their date of birth and what month it is. Only correct answers attract credit.	**0** = Answers both questions correctly. **1** = Answers one question correctly. **2** = Answers neither question correctly.
1c LOC commands: Ask the patient to open and close their eyes; then to grip and release the non-paretic hand or move their feet up and down if hands cannot be moved. If no response to command is seen, the task should be demonstrated.	**0** = Performs both tasks correctly. **1** = Performs one task correctly. **2** = Performs neither task correctly.
2 Best gaze:	**0** = Normal. **1** = Partial gaze palsy. Abnormal gaze in one or both eyes. **2** = Forced deviation, or total gaze paresis.

TABLE 5.6 NIH scale (*Continued*)

Instructions	Scale definition
3 Visual: Extinction receives a score of 1.	**0** = No visual loss. **1** = Partial hemianopia. **2** = Complete hemianopia. **3** = Bilateral hemianopia (blind including cortical blindness).
4 Facial palsy: 'Show me your teeth' or 'Raise eyebrows and close eyes'.	**0** = Normal symmetrical movement. **1** = Minor paralysis (flattened nasolabial fold, asymmetry on smiling). **2** = Partial paralysis (total or near total paralysis of lower face). **3** = Complete paralysis of one or both sides (absence of facial movement in the upper and lower face).
5 Motor arm: Score each arm individually	**0** = No drift, limb held at 90° (or 45°) for full 10 seconds. **1** = Limb drifts down before full 10 seconds; does not hit bed or other support. **2** = Some effort against gravity, limb cannot be elevated or maintained at 90° (or 45°), drifts down to bed but has some effort against gravity. **3** = No effort against gravity, limb falls. **4** = No movement. **9** = Amputation, joint fusion explain:
5a. Left arm **5b. Right arm**	
6 Motor leg: Score each leg individually	**0** = No drift, leg holds 30 degrees position for full five seconds. **1** = Drift, leg falls by the end of the five-second period but does not hit bed. **2** = Some effort against gravity; leg falls to bed by five seconds, but has some effort against gravity. **3** = No effort against gravity, leg falls to bed immediately. **4** = No movement. **9** = Amputation, joint fusion explain:
6a. Left leg **6b. Right leg**	

(*Continued*)

TABLE 5.6 NIH scale (*Continued*)

Instructions	Scale definition
7 Limb ataxia:	**0** = Absent **1** = Present in one limb **2** = Present in two limbs If present, is ataxia in right arm 1 = Yes 2 = No 9 = amputation or joint fusion, explain _____ Left arm 1 = Yes 2 = No 9 = amputation or joint fusion, explain _____ Right leg 1 = Yes 2 = No 9 = amputation or joint fusion, explain _____ Left leg 1 = Yes 2 = No 9 = amputation or joint fusion, explain _____
8 Sensory:	**0** = Normal; no sensory loss. **1** = Mild to moderate sensory loss; patient feels pinprick is less sharp or is dull on the affected side; or there is a loss of superficial pain with pinprick but patient is aware he/she is being touched. **2** = Severe to total sensory loss; patient is not aware of being touched in the face, arm, and leg.
9 Best language:	**0** = No dysphasia, normal. **1** = Mild to moderate dysphasia. **2** = Severe dysphasia. **3** = Mute, global aphasia.
10 Dysarthria	**0** = Normal. **1** = Mild to moderate; patient slurs at least some words and, at worst, can be understood with some difficulty. **2** = Severe (unintelligible speech). **9** = Intubated or other physical barrier, explain _____.
11 Extinction and inattention:	**0** = No abnormality. **1** = Visual, tactile, auditory, spatial, or personal inattention or extinction to bilateral simultaneous stimulation in one of the sensory modalities. **2** = Profound hemi-inattention or hemi-inattention to more than one modality.

INITIAL BEDSIDE EVALUATION
History
Anosognosia and collateral history

The value of clinical history is paramount but this is not always available, due to the fact that stroke often impairs cognition or causes dysphasia. Often the patient can communicate and narrate past events but lacks the ability to be aware of deficits and this may be due to *anosognosia*, a neglect seen with right hemisphere involvement. A collateral source of history is invaluable in this setting. In fact, availability of clinical history supportive of stroke has been reported to even increase the sensitivity for detecting strokes on unenhanced CT without reducing specificity.[2]

Is it definitely a stroke?

There are numerous stroke mimics. Table 5.7 presents a few important differential diagnoses that need to be considered. These will be reviewed in detail in Chapter 6.

The new tissue-based definition of TIA is *'transient episode of neurologic dysfunction caused by focal brain, spinal cord, or retinal ischaemia, without acute infarction'.* Infarction, i.e., tissue injury, is the defining feature here rather than the arbitrary time limit of 24 hours. TIA will be discussed in more detail in Chapter 7.

Ischaemic stroke or haemorrhage?

Headache and the presence of rapidly deteriorating and generally severe symptoms are more commonly seen with intracerebral haemorrhage. The value of clinical history in identifying this is limited and superseded by computed tomography, which is highly sensitive for the diagnosis of haemorrhage in the acute setting.[3]

Is there a clear onset time within the window for thrombolytic therapy?

The onset of stroke is sudden and the time of onset is the first aspect in the clinical history that should be identified, whether from the patient or observers.

TABLE 5.7 Differential diagnoses in acute stroke

Migraine
Other types of intracranial hemorrhage
Head trauma
Brain tumor
Todd's palsy (paresis, aphasia, neglect, etc., after a seizure episode)
Functional deficit (conversion reaction)
Systemic infection
Toxic-metabolic disturbances (hypoglycemia, acute renal failure, hepatic insufficiency, exogenous drug intoxication)

TABLE 5.8 Key areas in the history for those potentially suitable for thrombolysis

The following must be answered YES:
1 Does the patient have symptoms of acute stroke?
2 Is there a measurable deficit on the NIH scale?
3 Was the patient previously independent?
4 Is there a clear time of onset within the last 270 minutes?
5 Has a CT brain scan since stroke onset excluded haemorrhage?
6 Have you and other trained specialist personally looked at the CT film?

The following must be answered NO:
1 Has the patient suffered head trauma or stroke within the last three months?
2 Has the patient undergone major surgery within the last two weeks?
3 Is there a history of intracranial haemorrhage?
4 Is the history suggestive of subarachnoid haemorrhage?
5 Is SBP > 185 mm Hg?
6 Is DBP > 110 mm Hg?
7 Has any antihypertensive treatment been used to attain the above limits?
8 Are the symptoms/signs minor or rapidly improving?
9 Has there been GI or urinary tract haemorrhage within the last 21 days?
10 Has there been an arterial puncture at a non-compressible site within the last seven days?
11 Was there a seizure at the time of the stroke onset?
12 Has the patient taken anticoagulants or heparin within the last 48 hours, with an increased PTT?

Symptoms with a definite sudden onset within the 'thrombolysis window' of 270 minutes (4.5 hours) should be managed as a medical emergency. The history here should be accurate but rapid and suitability for thrombolytic treatment explored in a careful manner. A recommended scheme for exploring possible contraindications to thrombolytic therapy is given in Table 5.8 and comprises six questions where the answer must be YES and 12 questions where the answer must be NO.

GENERAL MEDICAL EXAMINATION

Stroke is a medical disorder and a general medical exam is imperative. This may reveal medical causes or even complications of stroke or might uncover a stroke mimic. An airway-breathing-circulation approach can be lifesaving and is highly recommended.

Primary stroke survey

1 *General*: Coma, vomiting, severe headache, hyperglycaemia, and a therapeutic anticoagulant state all point to a haemorrhagic cause of stroke.
2 *BP*: Stroke patients tend to be hypertensive and this may be a protective response to help maintain cerebral perfusion. However, significant hypertension

is associated with worse outcome and with haemorrhage extension and may require treatment. Very high blood pressure is a contraindication to thrombolytic therapy for ischaemic stroke and it is also important to monitor for management purposes (discussed later).

3 *Temp (T)*:   Temperature does not tend to be elevated in acute stroke and a high fever would suggest sepsis, either as a cause of the neurological deficit or in association with the stroke.

4 *Pulse*:   Assessment is important, as an irregularly irregular rate with an associated pulse deficit would point to AF and an embolic stroke. Absent pulses may be seen in Takayasu's arteritis (the 'pulseless disease'), which may present as stroke. Absent right-sided pulses indicate aortic dissection, which often mimics stroke.

Neurological examination

This is the cornerstone of stroke assessment and may allow lesion localisation, although a full neurological assessment is generally not required before thrombolytic therapy for example where assessment of the NIHSS may suffice. It must however be performed at some stage during the early hours of admission.

General signs

1 *Consciousness*:
   – reduced with damage to bifrontal or bithalamic regions or brainstem reticular activating system
   – hyperalertness is seen with alcohol/barbiturate withdrawal or psychiatric disease

2 *Neck stiffness*:
   – with the patient lying flat, the examiner slips a hand under the occiput and flexes the neck passively in a gentle manner until the chin is brought up to reach the chest wall
   – meningism due to meningeal irritation from infection or subarachnoid haemorrhage causes painful spasm of the neck extensors and thus resistance to neck flexion

3 *Kernig's sign*:
   – useful if meningitis is suspected
   – flex each hip in turn and attempt to straighten the knee while keeping the hip flexed (limited by hamstring spasm secondary to an inflammatory exudates around lumbar spinal roots)

Higher centres

1 *Handedness*: 94% of right-handed people and 50% of left-handed people have a dominant left hemisphere; the dominant hemisphere controls language and mathematical function

2   *Orientation* should be tested in ascending difficulty
    – *person*: 'What is your name'?
    – *place*: 'Where are you just now'?
    – *time*: 'What is the date (day, month, year)'?

Language

1   A laconic, seemingly disorientated, or mute patient would raise concern, and a detailed assessment of comprehension should be performed. For example, ask the patient to 'touch your chin, then your nose and then your ear'. **Receptive (posterior) or Wernicke's dysphasia** may be discovered here. This is caused by damage to the posterior part of the first temporal gyrus (Wernicke's area), and the patient cannot understand the spoken (auditory dysphasia) or the written word (alexia).

2   In the non-chatty patient, encourage flow of speech in an endeavour to detect *expressive* difficulties. Ask: 'Could you tell me where you live and how you would get home from here'? Expressive (anterior) or Broca's dysphasia may be revealed by such a simple question. This is caused by a lesion in the posterior dominant third frontal gyrus; the patient can understand, but speech is non-fluent and produced with great frustration with malformed words such as 'spoot' for 'spoon'.

3   *Articulation* is tested by asking the patient to repeat 'British constitution', 'baby hippopotamus', or 'West Register Street'. Difficulty denotes *dysarthria* due to incoordination or weakness of the musculature of speech. Dysarthria can be *spastic* or *flaccid*. Possible pathologies related to stroke comprise:
    a   Pseudobulbar palsy: the most common cause is bilateral cerebrovascular accidents of the internal capsule and involvement in lesions of IX, X, and XII; this results in slurred, monotonous, 'Donald Duck' speech; bilateral spasticity with positive Babinski can also be seen
    b   Bulbar palsy: implying bilateral LMN lesions of IX, X, and XII, caused by brainstem infarction and resulting in speech with nasal character
    c   Cerebellar disease causing ataxia of the speech muscles, resulting in slurring (as if drunk).

4   Ask the patient to *name two objects* such as a pen or a watch. Remember that the word stethoscope may be 'all Greek' to some, so avoid using it. **Nominal dysphasia** renders the patient unable to name objects and occurs with a lesion in the dominant posterior temporoparietal area. It also occurs in the recovery phase from any dysphasia and therefore has doubtful localising value.

5   Test *repetition* by asking the patient to repeat the above phrases or longer sentences; more traditional internists will command *'Repeat the phrase "no ifs, ands, or buts"'*. Inability to perform this task may be due to articulation problems (as above) or **conductive dysphasia**. This results from a lesion in the arcuate fasciculus or other fibres linking Wernicke's and Broca's areas; patients fail to repeat sentences but fluency and comprehension are adequate. Repitition helps assess

speech in laconic patients giving one-word answers in the history and may reveal any of the four types of dysphasia.

6   In order to complete language testing, ask the patient to *read* and *write*. Difficulty in reading (dyslexia) may be seen in expressive, receptive, conductive, or nominal dysphasia. Difficulty in writing (dysgraphia) is seen in expressive and conductive dysphasia. Dyslexia without agraphia implies lesion in the dominant occipital lobe and/or the splenium of the corpus callosum.

7   Acalculia can be diagnosed by asking the patient to perform some straightforward calculations (e.g., 'What is 4 + 9; 4 × 8; 27 − 18'?).

8   Agraphia should raise suspicion for exotic entities that could impress your consultant if diagnosed, and you should ask the patient to name individual fingers and test the ability to perform basic calculations. *Finger agnosia* is the inability to carry out this task and is part of **Gerstman's syndrome** (acalculia, agraphia, left-right confusion, and finger agnosia), which results from lesions of the angular gyrus of the dominant parietal lobe.

Neglect

These can be sensory, spatial, or motor and are more common with non-dominant (right) hemisphere lesions, especially when involving the parietal lobe.

1   *Sensory neglects* are tested for by looking for extinction to double simultaneous stimulation and localises to the occipito-parietal region.

2   *Spatial neglects* can be formally tested for by clock drawing.

3   *Motor neglects* that occur when one part of the body is underused, in the absence of overt weakness or loss of sensation.

4   *Neglect of the disease process* (anosognosia in Greek) is a deficit seen in non-dominant parietal strokes and should be uncovered as soon as asking the patient how they are.

Dyspraxias

These can be orofacial, constructional, or dressing and may be due to parietal lobe or prefrontal cortex strokes and can be tested by simple questions:

'Can you press your tongue against the inside of each cheek (against my hand, with a closed mouth)'?

'Can you show me how you would play the piano'?

'Can you do these buttons up'?

Frontal lobe dysfunction

Despite the large size of the frontal lobe and its common involvement in stroke, clinical frontal dysfunction is rather rare in stroke, possibly due to a volume effect. The presence of primitive reflexes (such as the grasp and palmomental reflexes); anosmia; gait apraxia (feet glued to the floor); disinhibition; abulia; and emotional disturbance are all suggestive of frontal damage. They all tend to indicate a recurrent, diffuse process, and the value of testing in the context of a new, sudden onset stroke-like event is limited.[4]

Cranial nerves

1 Olfactory (CN I): practically not tested in the setting of acute stroke
2 Optic (CN II):
   a Test *acuity* in each eye; this can be undertaken formally by using a Snellen chart held at 6 m from patient or by asking the patient to count fingers in front of each eye with spectacles on; alternatively, the patient is asked to read reasonably sized text; in reality, a simple question (*'How is your eyesight'?*) suffices for the observant clinician. Acuity may suffer in occipital lobe infarction.
   b *Visual fields* should be examined with the examiner's head being level with the patient's head; a red-tipped hat pin (for the keen) or two moving fingers should be brought into each visual field quadrangle. Classically, *homonymous hemianopia* may result from lesions of the optic tract to the occipital cortex; *upper quadrant homonymous hemianopia* is due to temporal lobe lesions; and *lower quadrant hemianopia* may complicate parietal lobe infarcts.
   c *Fundoscopy* should be performed; papilloedema, cholesterol emboli, chronic hypertensive changes, or diabetic changes may be readily identified by the experienced eye.
3 Oculomotor (CN III), trochlear (CN IV), and abducens (CN VI)
   a *Pupils:*
   Inspect for size and symmetry and test response to light, direct and consensual. Are they equal? Is there obvious anisocoria? Remember, a pupil can be either large and poorly constrictive or small and poorly dilating. Light induces pupil constriction, and if anisocoria is more marked in bright light, this raises suspicion of a deficit in the constriction apparatus (e.g., CN III lesion). The contrary is true for anisocoria that becomes more apparent in a darker room, and a deficit in the sympathetic pathway may be the culprit. Of course, carotid dissection should be considered as a differential diagnosis of anisocoria, especially in patients complaining of neck pain or in those who look Marfanoid. Bilaterally pinpoint pupils may occur with raised intracranial pressure or with bilateral pontine lesions.
   Test accommodation, which may be impaired in isolation with cortical blindness or midbrain lesions (syphilis may also be the culprit here; 'prostitute's pupil' accommodates but does not react to light).
   b *Eye movements:*
   Ask patient to follow your finger moving in an 'H' pattern and observe carefully for failure of movement in any direction, indicating ocular muscle involvement. Always check with the patient whether there is diplopia: covering the defective eye makes the lateral, pale, false image disappear. Abnormal eye movement and diplopia may be due to III, IV, or VI deficits.

Observe for an abnormality of conjugate gaze. Brainstem lesions cause ipsilateral whereas frontal lobe lesions cause contralateral paralysis of horizontal conjugate gaze. Deviation of the eyes to one side may result from lesions in the contralateral brainstem. A stroke affecting the dorsal pons may result in the peculiar one-and-a-half syndrome, whereby there is a horizontal gaze palsy when looking to one side plus impaired adduction when looking the other side.

c   *Nystagmus:*
Phenytoin, alcohol, and other toxins may cause both horizontal and vertical nystagmus, so this should be considered before drawing any premature conclusions.

Test for nystagmus by asking the patient to follow your finger out to 30° from the centre, as almost everyone will get nystagmus at the extremes of gaze. The direction of the nystagmus is defined as that of the fast movement.

Horizontal nystagmus may be due to vestibular, cerebellar, or more rarely medial longitudinal fasciculus lesions. The latter could be vascular in the old and can cause internuclear ophthalmoplegia, where there is nystagmus in the abducting eye and failure of adduction of the other. Such a finding in a young patient should raise suspicion of MS, although vascular causes may be responsible in the elderly.

Vertical nystagmus points to a brainstem lesion, whether midbrain or floor of fourth ventricle (when upbeat) or foramen magnum (when downbeat).

4   Trigeminal (CN V)
   a   Test light touch sensation on each side of the patient's forehead while asking if the two stimuli felt the same on both sides. This should be repeated on the cheek and on the chin. (NB. The superficial cervical plexus is responsible for sensation at the angle of the jaw).
   b   The above procedure should be repeated applying light pressure with a pin.
   c   Although not done routinely, the corneal reflex may be of value in the unconscious or uncooperative patient.
   d   The motor division of the trigeminal nerve should be tested by testing jaw opening and jaw closing.

5.   Facial (CN VII)
   a   Have the patient close his or her eyes tightly. Observe whether the lashes are buried equally on the two sides and whether you can open either eye manually. Then have the patient look up and wrinkle the forehead; note whether the two sides are equally wrinkled. Have the patient smile, and observe whether one side of the face is activated more quickly or more completely than the other.
   b   The pattern of facial weakness can help differentiate between central and peripheral lesions. When one entire side of the face is weak, the lesion is usually peripheral. With a central lesion (such as a stroke in one cerebral hemisphere), the forehead muscles are often spared because the portion of

the facial nerve nucleus supplying innervation to the forehead typically gets input from the motor strips of both cerebral hemispheres. The portion of the facial nerve nucleus innervating the lower face does not have the same bilateral input; its input is predominantly from the contralateral cortex.

6 Auditory/vestibular (CN VIII)

   a Ask *'Have you noticed any recent problems with your hearing'*?

   b Each ear should be tested separately with finger rubbing or whispering, while distracting the other ear. The Weber and Rhinne tests could be done for completeness in an attempt to characterise the hearing deficit as conductive or sensorineural.

   c In theory, a stroke involving the anterior inferior cerebellar artery (AICA) and thus the branching labyrinthine artery may cause unilateral deafness, but this is rarely encountered in practice. A basilar artery occlusion may involve both AICAs and thus lead to deafness among other neurological deficits.

   d A peripheral lesion is more frequently responsible for unilateral hearing deficits. Ischaemic cranial neuropathy and syphilis should be considered, among other causes of mononeuritis, which tend to be abrupt and thus mimic stroke.

7 Glossopharyngeal (CN IX) and vagus (CN X)

   a Ask the patient to open their mouth and say 'ah' and look for asymmetry in the movement of the posterior soft palate. The uvula points to the normal side.

   b The gag reflex is of limited value, as it is absent in the elderly and is sometimes difficult to interpret. It is tested by touching each side of the posterior pharynx with a spatula (CN IX is the afferent and CN X the efferent component of this reflex).

   c Swallowing should be tested by asking the patient to swallow a small amount of water, and regurgitation or any coughing should be noted.

   d Lateral medullary infarction (seen with vertebral or posterior inferior cerebellar artery lesions) may cause glossopharyngeal and vagus deficits.

8 Accessory (CN XI)

   Place your hand on the left side of the chin and say *'Turn your head against my hand'.* (NB. The right sternocleidomastoid turns the head to the left).

   Then say *'Shrug your shoulders up'* and remember to palpate the trapezius muscles while attempting to push the shoulders down.

   A central deficit would produce ipsilateral sternocleidomastoid weakness but contralateral trapezius weakness (i.e., weakness of shoulder elevation and weakness of head rotation toward the same side).

9 Hypoglossal (CN XII)

   a Say *'Stick out your tongue'* and inspect for wasting and fasciculations.

   b It is important to remember that the tongue (like the face and palate) is innervated bilaterally, so unilateral upper motor neuron deficits often cause no deviation but may result in an immobile tongue. A unilateral lower motor neuron lesion, on the other hand, makes the tongue deviate to the side of the lesion (i.e., the weaker, affected side).

c   In any case, ask the patient to move their tongue rapidly from side to side and push it against the left cheek from inside the mouth while you push against it from outside.

d   It is important to remember that the combination of bilateral UMN involvement of CN IX, X, and XII may be seen with bilateral internal capsule involvement, an entity known as *pseudobulbar palsy*. Other causes comprise multiple sclerosis and motor neuron disease; these present differently to stroke. In pseudobulbar palsy, the tongue appears spastic and the patient's dysarthria is also spastic.

e   Fasciculations and a nasal speech on a par with an absent gag reflex are seen in LMN lesions of CN IX, X, and XI, resulting in *bulbar palsy*. Brainstem infarction can cause this, along with Guillain-Barré and poliomyelitis.

Gait

1   Following careful observation of patient's casual gait, ask them to '*Walk with one foot in front of the other*'. Staggering towards the affected side would betray a cerebellar lesion, whether ischaemic or haemorrhagic. A wide-based gait betrays a drunken state!

Romberg's sign is a sensory system testing but it is recommended that it is examined with gait for convenience purposes. A negative (or false positive) Romberg's sign confirms cerebellar or vestibular dysfunction; ask '*Stand with your feet together*' and then '*Shut your eyes*' while ensuring you are ready to prevent an unsteady patient from falling. Profound unsteadiness when the eyes are open suggests cerebellar disease or vestibular dysfunction. The test is positive when unsteadiness is worsened by eye closure and denotes proprioceptive loss in the lower limbs.

2   When slapping of the feet accompanies a wide-based gait, a posterior column lesion may be the culprit.

3   If the patient's feet appear 'glued' to the floor while attempting to walk, suspect the *apraxic gait* denoting prefrontal lobe damage.

4   The scissoring gait of *spastic paraparesis* should be readily identified as should the *high stepping gait* of foot drop. These are seldom seen in acute stroke.

Motor system

1   *Inspection and palpation* of the muscle bulk should be done, as part of a complete neurological examination, aiming to detect atrophy and fasciculations. These are unlikely to be encountered in the acute setting. Abrasions and injuries restricted to one side may well betray the leg that 'gave way', i.e., the hemiparetic limb and observation can therefore be invaluable.

2   *Tone* is assessed by passive manipulation of a 'floppy' limb and is tested at wrist and elbow in the upper limbs and at knees and ankles in the lower limbs. Clonus

should also be tested for by rapid dorsiflexion with a knee bent and a thigh externally rotated. Tone, which is classically increased in central lesions and reduced in peripheral ones, may be found to be increased in the acute setting, especially in deep white matter lesions. Other pathologies may always become apparent, and a first presentation of Parkinson's may be revealed by co-incidentally discovering cogwheel rigidity.

3 *Power*

   a To test **drift**, ask '*Shut your eyes and stretch your arms out and turn your palms upwards*'. Watch for five to 10 seconds to see if either arm drifts down and pronates. A unilateral pronator drift suggests an UMN lesion on the same side. This is because of the fact that the UMN pattern of weakness causes supination of the upper limbs to be weaker than pronation. An abnormal searching movement may be seen with loss of proprioception (also known as pseudoathetosis). Upward movement may suggest cerebellar or parietal lobe deficit.

   b **Strength** is tested in upper (at shoulder, elbow, wrist, and fingers) and lower limbs (at hip, knee, ankle, and tarsal joint). Muscle strength should be graded using the Medical Research Council scale (*see* Table 5.9).

   c The pattern of weakness in UMN lesions involves extensors that are weaker than flexors in arms and extensors stronger than flexors in legs.

4 *Reflexes*

   a The biceps (C5, C6), triceps (C7, C8), brachioradialis (C5, C6), and finger (C8) jerks normally cause contraction of the muscle, resulting in forearm flexion at the elbow; forearm extension at the elbow; forearm flexion; and slight flexion of all fingers, respectively.

   b The knee (L3, L4), ankle (S1, S2), and plantar (L5, S1, and S2) reflexes normally cause knee extension, plantar flexion, and a flexor plantar response, respectively. When the plantar response is abnormal (extensor), this is known as Babinski's sign.

   c Reflexes are best elicited when the patient is relaxed and may be reinforced by distracting manoeuvres

   d There is a grading system for the deep tendon reflexes, but it is not universally adopted. In reality, comparison of the two sides and a description such as 'present', 'absent', 'increased', or 'reduced' would suffice.

TABLE 5.9 The MRC scale for grading muscle strength

0 = no contraction
1 = visible muscle twitch but no movement
2 = weak contraction, capable of rolling on bed but insufficient to overcome gravity
3 = weak contraction able to overcome gravity
4 = weak contraction able to overcome some resistance
5 = normal; able to overcome full resistance

5 *Coordination*

   a Coordination testing is sometimes erroneously referred to as cerebellar testing. It is clear that the cerebellum plays an integral part in the production of coordinated movements, but strength and sensation are as important.

   b The **finger-to-nose testing** should detect any intention tremor or past-pointing, as seen in cerebellar disease.

   c **Rapidly alternating movements** can be tested for by asking the patient to pronate and supinate each hand on the dorsum if the other. Dysdiadochokinesis is Greek for clumsy movement and occurs in cerebellar disease. Internal capsule infarction may also impair rapidly alternating movements, as may extrapyramidal disorders such as Parkinson's disease.

   d **Rebound** and **overshoot** may be impaired due to hypotonia in cerebellar disease.

   e The **heel-shin**, **toe-finger**, and **foot tapping** tests are performed in the lower limbs.

Sensory system

1 Prior to testing the *primary sensory modalities*, ask the patient whether they feel any numbness or anything else different. Then test **light touch** (which travels in dorsal columns) using a piece of cotton wool, trying to avoid stroking the skin. **Pinprick** comes next (with **temperature** testing only undertaken in special circumstances and by keen physicians); both of these run in spinothalamic tracts. **Vibration** (using a 128 Hz tuning fork) and **proprioception** run in dorsal columns and should also be tested (bearing in mind that abnormalities in vibration sense usually suggest peripheral neuropathy).

2 Testing for **cortical sensory loss** comprises testing for two-point discrimination, agraphaesthesia, astereognosis, and atopographia and in reality are only done by those with a special interest in neurology.

Cardiovascular examination

Although stroke causes abnormal neurological signs, its underlying cause may frequently be identified by careful examination of the cardiovascular system.

Murmurs and *added heart sounds* raise the possibility of concurrent cardiac pathology, such as acute coronary syndrome and rarer entities such as atrial myxoma as underlying aetiologies. Malfunctioning valves, particularly in conjunction with atrial fibrillation, raise the possibility of ischaemic stroke secondary to embolisation.

The *carotid arteries* should be auscultated for bruits suggesting stenosis, but imaging of vertebral and carotid arteries remains essential. Other facial pulses can be palpated in an attempt to reveal compensatory ECA flow secondary to ICA occlusion, but the overall value of this is questionable and we do not generally recommend it in the acute setting.

Dermatological examination

This may appear less relevant in acute stroke but should be done as part of the general medical examination. It may help identify interesting underlying pathologies or rare causes of stroke.

A reactive paraneoplastic erythema, for example, may point to malignancy, which is a pro-coagulant state. Tar staining may betray the tobacco enthusiast, who would essentially be at high risk of stroke.

Splinter haemorrhages and Janeway lesions may be seen with infective endocarditis. Xanthelasmata and tendon xanthomata suggest hypercholesterolaemia Livedo reticularis is seen in the rare Sneddon's syndrome and a malar rash may betray the hypercoagulable state of SLE.

Striae in a slim, tall, young patient with high-arched palate, crowded teeth, and pectus carinatum or excavatum should raise suspicion of Marfan's. Among other things, such patients may present with carotid artery dissection, but lacking risk factors, suspecting primary arteriopathy (whether Marfan's or pseudoxanthoma) would be very reasonable.

Initial investigations
Brain imaging

Brain imaging is essential for any acute stroke, and computed tomography (CT) is the standard immediate study and should be performed as soon as possible. Magnetic resonance imaging is more sensitive; these techniques are discussed in more detail in Chapter 10.

Blood tests

A complete full blood (including platelet) count, erythrocyte sedimentation rate, blood glucose level, thrombin time and partial thromboplastin time, lipid levels, and acute phase protein measurement, such as C-reactive protein and renal function, should be checked. Blood cultures should be also performed in a patient with pyrexia.

FURTHER EVALUATION OF THE STROKE PATIENT
Post thrombolytic therapy

Admission to a specialised acute stroke unit is imperative and has been shown to be highly beneficial. Nursing patients who have received thrombolytic therapy is intense and comprises cardiac monitoring for 24 hours and frequent blood pressure and neurological monitoring. Repeat CT brain scanning is essential at 24 hours post-thrombolysis administration in order to exclude haemorrhagic transformation in an area of infarction.

All stroke patients

Physical evaluation

The patient should be reevaluated to assess whether there is any change in their neurological state. If the neurological exam was not done thoroughly on admission, this should be done in the first 24 hours. Physical examination should also be thorough and complete.

Speech and language assessment and physiotherapy review should be performed within the first 24 hours.

Further imaging

An MRI may be necessary, especially when no cause of the presenting deficit has been found. Cerebral angiography, either with CT or MR, should be considered in those with intracerebal haemorrhage.

Cardiac investigations

An ECG may successfully identify patients who have atrial fibrillation (AF) as a source of emboli, and monitoring for the first 24 hours is currently recommended practice. Monitoring for longer than 24 hours may need to be undertaken in order to identify intermittent paroxysms of AF. An ECG may also reveal changes of underlying ischaemic heart disease.

A transthoracic echocardiogram (TTE) is required in all patients with embolic stroke, especially in the young or older but atypical patient. TTE can readily identify left ventricular thrombi in patients with heart failure, although transoesophageal echocardiography (TOE) is more sensitive and better at excluding aortic atheromatous disease, atrial septal aneurysm, and patent foramen ovale. It is, however, a more invasive and demanding procedure.

Haematological investigations

In addition to the routine bloods, more specialised blood tests may be required, including a thrombophilia screen, assessment of antiphospholipid antibodies, fibrinogen, urate, syphilis, Lyme disease, and HIV serology.

Vascular studies

If the clinical picture suggests an anterior circulation stroke, the carotid arteries (extra- and intracranial) and the middle (MCA) and anterior (ACA) cerebral arteries should be considered as culprits. Duplex ultrasound of the neck and transcranial Doppler (TCD) of the intracranial vessels can help identify culprit stenoses and are discussed in more detail in Chapter 12.

Doppler scanning of the vertebral and subclavian arteries may demonstrate atheromatous disease and potentially uncover the aetiology of posterior circulation events. The direction of flow within the vertebral artery can be assessed and this may suggest proximal obstruction.

TCD may be used for detecting high-intensity transient signals (HITS) and these correspond to clinically silent microemboli passing through the beam of the ultrasound probe. These may suggest a proximal source of emboli such as an unstable carotid plaque. The role of microemboli detection in routine clinical practice remains controversial but is the focus of ongoing research and is discussed further in Chapter 10.

If further investigation is necessary, CT or MR angiography may be helpful in examining vertebral and carotid arteries, although their origin in the neck is sometimes more difficult to define.

REFERENCES

1. Kidwell CS, Starkman S, Eckstein M, *et al*. Identifying Stroke in the Field: Prospective Validation of the Los Angeles Prehospital Stroke Screen (LAPSS) *Stroke*. 2000; **31**: 71–6.
2. Mullins ME, Lev MH, Schellingerhout D, *et al*. Influence of availability of clinical history on detection of early stroke using unenhanced CT and diffusion-weighted MR imaging. *American Journal of Roentgenology*. 2002; **179**: 223–228
3. Beauchamp NJ, Bryan RN. Neuroimaging of stroke. In: Welch KM, Caplan LR, Reis DJ, *et al*., editors. *Primer on Cerebrovascular Diseases*. Academic Press; 1997: 599.
4. Bogousslavsky J. Frontal lobe dysfunction in cerebrovascular disease. *Schweizer Archiv für Neurologie und Psychiatrie*. 2003; **154**(2): 59–65.

FURTHER READING

* Douglas G, Nicol F, Roberston C. *Macleod's Clinical Examination*. 12th international ed. Churchill Livingstone; 2009.
* Talley N, O'Connor S. *Clinical Examination: a systematic guide to physical diagnosis*. 6th international ed. Churchill Livingstone; 2009.

CHAPTER 6

Evidence-based management

INTRODUCTION

There are several rational therapeutic targets in the early hours after onset of acute stroke. Infarct volume increases in the first few hours after ischaemic stroke, with the ischaemic penumbra gradually being subsumed into the area of infarction. The penumbra is the region of the brain where blood supply is significantly reduced but energy metabolism is maintained because of collateral flow. If blood flow is swiftly restored, some penumbral tissue may be saved. This is the aim of reperfusion therapy. However, during the time lag to reperfusion, cellular metabolism becomes anaerobic leading to acidosis, and sodium-potassium transporters become dysfunctional, causing a rise in intracellular osmolarity and cytotoxic oedema. Intracellular calcium concentration increases, which enhances injury through activation of lipase, protease, and free radical generation. Furthermore, even if reperfusion occurs, the penumbra is vulnerable to the effects of reperfusion injury. Altering such processes is the aim of neuroprotection therapy. In the context of intracerebral haemorrhage, it has recently been recognised that early haemorrhage growth can occur and that this is associated with worse outcome. Thus, for both ischaemic and haemorrhagic stroke, there are therapeutic targets but they exist only in the early hours after stroke. Urgent diagnosis, investigation, and treatment are therefore vital. All patients are at risk of a further stroke, and reducing this risk is also a key aim.

CURRENT ACUTE MANAGEMENT STRATEGIES

Potential effective treatments for acute stroke include control of physiological variables, strategies to reperfuse an ischaemic area, measures to reduce growth of primary intracerebral haemorrhage (haemostatic therapy, currently unproven), protection of the vulnerable, yet salvageable, ischaemic penumbra (neuroprotectant therapy, currently unproven), and surgery. All patients must be offered care in a dedicated acute stroke unit, which saves lives and significantly improves functional outcomes.

Stroke unit care

A stroke unit is an area and environment of organised and multidisciplinary care which ensures access to specialist medical, nursing, and allied staff and treatment. Randomised controlled trials show that patients have better functional outcome and better survival if cared for in a stroke unit compared to a general ward or staying at home.[1] The mechanism of this benefit is not fully established but is likely to be due to both better medical, nursing, and rehabilitation care.

Control of physiological variables

Arterial hypertension occurs in as many as 80% of patients following acute stroke and is associated with a poor outcome.[2] However, falls in blood pressure may lead to infarct extension because of impaired cerebrovascular autoregulation following acute stroke and there is some evidence that a U-shaped relationship exists (arterial hypotension is also associated with a poor outcome). Routine lowering of blood pressure is not recommended by current UK and pan-European current consensus guidelines. Blood pressure should be cautiously lowered in the presence of hypertensive encephalopathy, aortic dissection, and severe cardiac failure if it is extremely high on repeated measurement (> 220 mm Hg systolic or > 120 mm Hg diastolic blood pressure). Some guidelines suggest that blood pressure be gradually lowered by a maximum of 20% of the mean arterial pressure to a target of 110 mm Hg if no known hypertension and to 125 mm Hg in the presence of a history of hypertension. This leaves a great deal of uncertainty in the majority of patients. Further, it is unclear whether prior antihypertensive therapy should be discontinued in the acute phase and at what thresholds of blood pressure we should intervene and the treatment targets that we should aim for. A recent large clinical trial evaluated the effect of treatment with candesartan, an angiotensin receptor antagonist in hypertensive acute stroke patients and found no evidence of benefit.[3] Other blood pressure-lowering strategies are being tested in separate trials; however, the current evidence does not support the routine treatment of moderately elevated blood pressure in the context of acute stroke.

Elevated blood glucose is common in the acute phase following ischaemic stroke and is associated with a poor outcome, regardless of the presence of pre-existing diabetes. In a recent systematic review and meta-analysis of non-diabetic patients, stress hyperglycaemia defined as blood glucose of greater than 6 or 7.1 mmol/L was strongly predictive of increased hospital mortality (RR 3.28, 95% CI 2.32–4.64) and poor functional outcome (RR 1.41, 95% CI 1.16–1.73). This may be because elevated blood glucose increases brain lactate production, which is associated with increased infarct size, may reduce the efficacy of thrombolytic therapy, and may increase the risk of haemorrhagic transformation of infarcted tissue. However, whether routine lowering of hyperglycaemia with insulin improves outcome after acute stroke is as yet unproven. Results from the recent GIST-UK (Glucose Insulin in Stroke) trial[4] were disappointing and showed no evidence of benefit for insulin therapy in terms of clinical outcome, although blood pressure and glucose levels were lowered by treatment. At present, current guidelines do not suggest routine lowering of blood sugar, although many use insulin titration in those with serum glucose of > 10 mmol/L. Avoidance of hypoglycaemia and hyperglycaemia are recommended.

Fever has also been associated with a poor outcome following acute stroke, possibly because of a detrimental effect on intracerebral metabolism, increased free radical production, or changes in blood-brain barrier function. It is again unclear whether treatment of pyrexia improves clinical outcome and trials are in progress to evaluate this. It is currently recommended to investigate fever and use anti-pyretic medication to lower body temperature when it occurs.

Intravenous thrombolytic therapy for acute ischaemic stroke

Thrombolytic therapy with tissue plasminogen activator (rt-PA) is the only licensed treatment for acute ischaemic stroke in Europe, where it must be administered within three hours of symptom onset. Evidence of benefit up to 4.5 hours after ictus is now established,[5] although the license is as yet unchanged. First evidence of efficacy was published in 1995 and license was granted for use in the United States in 1997 and in Europe (on a conditional basis) in 2002. Uptake of thrombolytic therapy remains poor in many countries. Contraindications for use of thrombolytic therapy in Europe are shown in Table 6.1.

A recent pooled meta-analysis[6] of the major thrombolytic therapy studies showed clear benefit for the treatment of ischaemic stroke. The analysis considered 2775 patients treated within six hours of ictus. The odds of favourable outcome (defined as no disability) were 2.8 (95% CI 1.8–9.5) for treatment within 90 minutes and 1.6 (95% CI 1.1–2.2) for treatment between 91 and 180 minutes. Benefit was still apparent for patients treated between 181 and 270 minutes (odds ratio 1.4, 95% CI 1.1–1.9). The rate of significant intracerebral haemorrhage was 5.9% in those treated with rt-PA compared to 1.1% in those treated with placebo, although not all of these were of clinical significance. Importantly, this risk of haemorrhage is already accounted for in the calculation of odds of favourable outcome. Thus, the chance of being free of handicap after stroke is increased nearly threefold by thrombolytic treatment if treated early and smaller but still significant benefits are seen up to 4.5 hours. The number needed to treat (NNT) to achieve an excellent outcome (and avert one case of death or dependency) following treatment is approximately 7 while the NNT to achieve a reduction in disability is estimated at approximately 3. The number needed to harm is approximately 30 and, for example, these figures compare favourably with those for thrombolytic therapy in acute MI. Recent data show that benefit does extend beyond 3 hours with increased the odds of an excellent outcome (OR 1.34, 1.02 to 1.76, p = 0.04) with an acceptably low rate of symptomatic intracerebral haemorrhage (2.4%)[7] provided treatment is given before 4.5 hours.

TABLE 6.1 Contraindication for use of rt-PA in ischaemic stroke

Specific contraindications for use of rt-PA in ischaemic stroke	General contraindication for any use of rt-PA
Evidence of intracranial haemorrhage	Significant bleeding disorder within past six months
Onset of symptoms > three hours from treatment or onset time unknown	Manifest or recent (< six months) severe bleeding
Age < 18 years or > 80 years	Known bleeding diathesis
Minor deficit or symptoms rapidly improving before start of infusion	Taking oral anti-coagulants
Severe stroke (NIHSS > 25, or severe stroke on brain imaging)	History of intracranial haemorrhage
Seizure at onset of stroke	Any history of CNS damage
Symptoms suggestive of subarachnoid haemorrhage	Recent (< 10 days) CPR
Platelet count < 100,000 per mm^3	Bacterial endocarditis or pericarditis
Heparin within past 48 hours and raised aPTT	Acute pancreatitis
Prior stroke within last three months	Ulcerative gastrointestinal disease during the last three months or known oesophageal varices or arterial/venous malformation
Prior stroke and concomitant diabetes	Neoplasm with increased bleeding risk
Systolic blood pressure > 185 or diastolic > 110 mm Hg or aggressive management required to reduce blood pressure to within these limits	Recent puncture of non-compressible blood vessel
	Major surgery or significant trauma within past three months
	Severe liver disease
	Obstetric delivery

Efficacy and safety of treatment in routine clinical practice has been confirmed by the Safe Implementation of Thrombolysis in Stroke-Monitoring (SITS-MOST) study.[6] This large registry of all patients treated within the terms of the license across Europe showed outcomes similar to the treatment arms of the randomised trials with low rates of symptomatic significant haemorrhage (Table 6.2). Mild systemic bleeding can of course occur and there is a risk of angio-oedema of approximately 1%, which is typically mild.

Risk factors for intracerebral haemorrhage following thrombolytic therapy include increasing age, extensive early infarct change on brain imaging, diabetes mellitus (DM), elevated blood glucose, DM and a history of previous stroke, and a low platelet count. Those with higher baseline stroke severity may also have a higher risk but equally may derive greatest benefit from treatment.

TABLE 6.2 Summary of outcomes in thrombolysis studies and the SITS register

	Mortality (at 3/12)	Independent (at 3/12)	S-ICH (Per SITS-MOST)*	S-ICH[†]
Trials	17.3%	49%	N/A	8.6%
SITS-MOST	11.3%	54.8%	1.7%	7.3%
Placebo	18.4%	30.2%	N/A	1.9%

* = Bleed large enough to cause symptoms and accompanying neurological deterioration.
† = Any bleed with any alteration in neurological status regardless of severity.

Intra-arterial thrombolysis/mechanical reperfusion

Intra-arterial thrombolysis involves direct catheterisation of an occluded artery and local administration of thrombolytic agents. This approach has been shown to be effective for middle cerebral artery (MCA) or basilar artery occlusion. In the PROACT II (Prolyse in Acute Cerebral Thromboembolism) trial,[8] where treatment was initiated within six hours of onset, reperfusion rates in those with confirmed MCA occlusion were significantly higher following intra-arterial thrombolysis with urokinase and intravenous heparin (66% compared to 18% in heparin treated controls, $p < 0.001$). Clinical outcomes were also significantly improved, with more patients living independently at day 90 (40% compared to 25% of controls, $p = 0.043$, relative risk reduction 58%).

Basilar artery occlusion carries a grave prognosis with a high mortality rate—perhaps in excess of 70%. While randomised controlled trial evidence are lacking, several case series have been published that suggest reduced mortality rates following intra-arterial thrombolysis, although outcomes are probably similar intra-arterial or intravenous treatment. The emphasis is therefore on urgent treatment using either modality.

Clot retrieval devices are in use in some centres but are not yet supported by definitive randomized controlled trial evidence.

Aspirin treatment

Aspirin has a modest but important effect in acute ischaemic stroke; a combined analysis of two large randomized controlled trials revealed nine fewer deaths or fatal strokes for every 1000 patients treated. It is generally advised to withhold aspirin therapy for 24 hours after thrombolytic therapy.

Anticoagulant therapy

Early anticoagulation has not been shown to yield benefit early after stroke. The small benefits in terms of improved outcome and fewer early recurrent strokes are offset by an increase in the number of those with subsequent symptomatic intracranial haemorrhage. It is of course an important preventative measure for DVT and for recurrent ischaemic stroke in some patients in the longer term.

Prophylaxis of venous thromboembolism

Those with intracerebral haemorrhage are not normally prescribed prophylactic doses of heparin in the very early stages (although practice does differ between countries and individuals). In those with ischaemic stroke, prophylactic doses of low molecular weight heparin, even if started early, are superior to unfractionated heparin in terms of reducing venous thromboembolism and do not appear to convey unacceptable haemorrhage risk.

Specific treatment for intracerebral haemorrhage

Supportive treatment is indicated as for all types of stroke. Rapid reversal of anticoagulation is required for anticoagulation-associated haemorrhage but otherwise there are no specific licensed treatments for the majority with spontaneous intracerebral haemorrhage.

Surgical treatment of acute stroke

Complete MCA infarction can be associated with massive brain oedema and increased intracranial pressure; the so-called malignant middle cerebral artery syndrome. When this occurs, mortality can be as high as 80% and medical therapy has little effect. Decompressive hemicraniectomy reduces the associated mortality and improves functional outcome in those aged under 60 years.[9] Compared to best medical treatment, numbers needed to treat to prevent death, severe disability, or moderate disability are 2, 2, and 4, respectively. Surgery has not yet been shown to be effective in unselected patients with ICH although is often considered to avoid or treat hydrocephalus in those with cerebellar haematoma and may be effective in those with peripheral lobar haematoma. Surgical treatment for those with raised intracranial pressure and hydrocephalus may be considered in those with acute stroke. Clinical trials are currently underway to further evaluate the role of surgery.

Summary of acute treatments

For ischaemic stroke, proven effective interventions are stroke unit care, aspirin, and reperfusion therapy with intravenous thrombolytic therapy. Intra-arterial thrombolysis is of benefit in a small subset of patients with large artery occlusion and ischaemic stroke. Beyond stroke unit care, there is no specific licensed treatment for ICH.

PREVENTION OF STROKE

Current preventative strategies include antiplatelet therapy and lipid-lowering therapy to prevent ischaemic stroke, anticoagulant therapy to prevent cardioembolic stroke, and blood pressure reduction to prevent all stroke subtypes. It is also recommended that patients undergo screening for and treatment of prevalent diabetes mellitus, smoking cessation therapy, and lifestyle modification.

Antiplatelet strategies

Aspirin is the only licensed strategy for the primary prevention of stroke. There are four main antiplatelet therapy regimens used to prevent recurrent stroke. These are aspirin, clopidogrel, dipyridamole, and the combination of aspirin and extended-release dipyridamole (Table 6.3).

Aspirin (acetylsalicylic acid) prevents platelet aggregation by irreversible inhibition of cyclooxygenase-1 (COX-1). The role of aspirin for primary prevention of cardiovascular disease is debated, although it may reduce the risk of first MI and of stroke in women. It will prevent up to a fifth of recurrent strokes, and most studies suggest an approximate relative risk reduction of 15% in comparison with placebo.[10]

Ticlopidine does reduce risk of vascular events compared to placebo and is probably similar to aspirin in terms of efficacy but is not licensed in the UK because of a risk of severe neutropenia and thrombotic thrombocytopenia.

The large CAPRIE trial compared clopidogrel monotherapy to aspirin in patients with symptomatic cardiovascular disease (recent stroke, MI, or symptomatic peripheral vascular disease).[11] Clopidogrel, an ADP receptor antagonist, gave a small but statistically significant reduction in the rate of the primary composite endpoint of ischaemic stroke, MI, or vascular death, predominantly driven by an effect in those with peripheral vascular disease. There were no differences between the drugs in terms of stroke rates and no differences in those who entered the trial because of previous stroke.

Dipyridamole, an adenosine reuptake inhibitor, is superior to placebo in terms of recurrent stroke prevention, but not in prevention of myocardial infarction or vascular death. It may have similar efficacy to aspirin but again without proven benefit in prevention of MI. This similar efficacy is at the cost of side effects such as headache. Aspirin and dipyridamole in combination are superior to placebo and to aspirin monotherapy. In the recent ESPRIT trial, the combination of aspirin and slow-release dipyridamole gave a significant reduction in the rate of vascular death or non-fatal stroke or MI compared to aspirin alone.[12]

Trials have shown that in the secondary prevention of stroke, dual therapy with clopidogrel and aspirin is no better than either alone. For example, the large CHARISMA trial[13] compared aspirin and clopidogrel therapy with aspirin alone, and approximately a quarter entered the trial because of previous cerebrovascular disease. Clopidogrel was no more effective than placebo in aspirin-treated patients in the entire cohort. In the secondary prevention cohort, there was a small reduction in the primary endpoint, a trend toward benefit in those who entered the trial on account of stroke, and all-cause stroke appeared lower in the population as a whole. However, these small benefits were countered by a near twofold increase in bleeding complications with combination therapy. In the MATCH trial,[14] no differences, apart from an increased bleeding rate with aspirin and clopidogrel, was seen between dual therapy and clopidogrel alone in those with recent stroke or TIA. The CARESS trial[15] compared the use of aspirin and clopidogrel with aspirin in patients with recently symptomatic > 50% carotid stenosis and microembolic signals. The number of microembolic signals was reduced by dual therapy and there was a strong trend towards a reduction in rate of stroke or TIA, although numbers were small.

The recent PRoFESS study[16] compared aspirin and dipyridamole with clopidogrel and there was no difference between the two treatment arms, although clopidogrel monotherapy was slightly better tolerated.

TABLE 6.3 Clinical trials of antiplatelet strategies for the prevention of stroke

Trial	Population	Primary endpoint	Intervention and primary endpoint rate
ATC* N = 10 000	Previous stroke/ TIA	Vascular event	Antiplatelet—18% Placebo—22% Reduction in odds of event with antiplatelet 22%, p < 0.0001
CAPRIE N = 19 185	Atherosclerotic vascular disease	Ischaemic stroke, MI, vascular death	Clopidogrel—5.32% Aspirin—5.83% Relative reduction in risk of event with clopidogrel 8.7%, 95% CI 0.3 to 16.5%
ESPRIT N = 2763	Previous TIA or minor stroke taking aspirin	Vascular death, stroke, MI, major bleeding complication	Dipyridamole—13% Placebo—16% Hazard ratio for event with dipyridamole 0.8, 95% CI 0.68 to 0.98
CHARISMA N = 15 603	Vascular disease or multiple risk factors treated with aspirin	Vascular death, MI or stroke.	Clopidogrel—6.8% Placebo—7.3% Relative reduction in risk of event with clopidogrel 0.93, 95% CI 0.83 to 1.05
MATCH N = 7599	Recent stroke or TIA treated with clopidogrel	Vascular death, stroke, MI, or rehospitalisation for an ischaemic event	Aspirin—15.7% Placebo—16.7% Relative reduction in risk of event with aspirin 6.4%, 95% CI –4.6% to 16.3%
PRoFESS N = 20 332	Previous ischaemic stroke or TIA	Recurrent stroke	Aspirin and dipyridamole—9% Clopidogrel—8% Hazard ratio for event with aspirin and dipyridamole 0.99, 95% CI 0.92 to 1.07

* = Antiplatelet Trialists Collaboration. TIA = transient ischaemic attack, MI = myocardial infarction. Abbreviated trial names are given and full references are found at the end of the chapter.

In summary, aspirin, clopidogrel, and dipyridamole monotherapy appear to provide similar efficacy in the secondary prevention of stroke. The combination of aspirin and clopidogrel poses unacceptable risks for little gain, except perhaps in certain high-risk subgroups. Aspirin and extended-release dipyridamole has been shown to be superior to aspirin in two studies, but recent data suggest this strategy offers similar yield to clopidogrel monotherapy, which is better tolerated. However, clopidogrel has not been shown to be superior to aspirin in the context of stroke prevention, either in the primary or secondary preventative setting. At present therefore, a reasonable strategy would be to employ aspirin and dipyridamole combination therapy, and where patients are intolerant to dipyridamole, to use clopidogrel monotherapy.

Anticoagulant therapy for non–cardioembolic stroke

There is no benefit above that of aspirin therapy from the use of warfarin in those with ischaemic stroke and no evidence of cardioembolic stroke. There may also be an increased haemorrhage rate and accordingly, anticoagulation is not recommended in this setting.

Statin/cholesterol-lowering therapy

Statin therapy is now an accepted strategy following ischaemic stroke. In a large meta-analysis of over 90 000 patients (mostly with manifest CHD) who were enrolled in statin trials, statin treatment significantly reduced the risk of incident stroke (OR 0.79, 95% CI 0.73–0.85).[16] Each 10% reduction in LDL cholesterol appears to afford an approximate 16% relative risk reduction for stroke, which is less than the reduction afforded for coronary heart disease. Interestingly, in the Heart Protection Study (HPS),[18] which enrolled over 20 000 patients with CHD or relevant risk factors and compared simvastatin 40 mg with placebo, the risk of first stroke was reduced by 25% (95% CI 15% to 34%, $p < 0.0001$) but the risk of recurrent stroke was unaffected. It was, however, reduced in the SPARCL trial,[19] where high-dose (80 mg) atorvastatin was used. High-dose lipid-lowering therapy is therefore justified in those with ischaemic stroke (Table 6.4).

An important consideration is the epidemiological link between low serum cholesterol and incidence of haemorrhagic stroke, which raises the possibility that statin therapy may increase risk of ICH. The SPARCL trial did show an increased risk of haemorrhagic stroke in those in the treatment arm (HR 1.67, 95% CI 1.09 to 2.56) and similar was found when data were combined with those from the HPS in a meta-analysis. However, the same meta-analysis revealed a much larger reduction in the risk of the more common recurrent ischaemic stroke and a reduction in the overall recurrent stroke burden.

In summary, statin therapy is clearly indicated and recommended as a preventative strategy in those who have suffered ischaemic stroke and high-dose

TABLE 6.4 Clinical trials of lipid lowering, antihypertensive, and anticoagulant therapy for the prevention of stroke

Trial	Population	Primary endpoint	Intervention and primary endpoint rate
Statin studies			
Meta-analysis N = 90 000	Varied across trials	Fatal or non-fatal stroke*	Statin therapy—2.7% Control—3.4% Odds ratio for event with statin therapy 0.79, 95% CI 0.73–0.85
HPS N = 20 536	Vascular disease or diabetes	Mortality	Simvastatin—12.9% Placebo—14.7% p = 0.0003
SPARCL N = 4731	Stroke or TIA	Fatal or non-fatal stroke	Atorvastatin 80 mg—11.2% Placebo—13.1% Hazard ratio for event with atorvastatin 0.84, 95% CI 0.71 to 0.99.
Blood pressure studies			
Meta-analysis # N = 15 527	Previous stroke or TIA	Fatal or non-fatal stroke	Active treatment—9% Control—11% Odds ratio for event with active blood pressure treatment 0.76, 95% CI 0.63–0.92
PROGRESS N = 6105	Previous stroke or TIA	Fatal or non-fatal stroke	Perindopril ± indapamide—10% Placebo—14% Relative reduction in risk of event with perindopril-based treatment 28%, 95% CI 17 to 38%
Anticoagulation studies			
European Atrial Fibrillation Trial	TIA or minor stroke	Death from vascular disease, stroke MI or systemic embolism	Anticoagulation—8% Placebo—17% Hazard ratio for event with anticoagulation 0.53, 95% CI 0.36 to 0.79
Other studies			
PROactive N = 5238	Type 2 diabetes and macrovascular disease	Mortality, non-fatal MI, stroke, or other major vascular event	Pioglitazone—20% Placebo—22% Hazard ratio for event with pioglitazone 0.9, 95% CI 0.8 to 1.02

* = results for the secondary stroke endpoint shown. # = results from secondary prevention meta-analysis shown. TIA = transient ischaemic attack, MI = myocardial infarction. Abbreviated trial names are given and full references are found at the end of the chapter.

lipid-lowering regimens are justified. There is little evidence to support routine use of statin therapy in those who have suffered ICH and have no other indication for their use.

Blood pressure–lowering therapy

Treatment of hypertension is of unequivocal benefit in reducing stroke risk in the primary prevention setting and evidence suggests that newer antihypertensive agents, such as amlodipine and angiotensin receptor blockers (ARBs), offer greater protection than 'older' atenolol and diuretic-based regimens.

Treatment of hypertension is also of benefit in the secondary prevention setting. For example, in a recent meta-analysis, odds of recurrent stroke were reduced by 24% (OR 0.76, 95% CI 0.63–0.92).[20] Interestingly, the strongest evidence exists for diuretic-based therapies, as opposed to ACE inhibitor or ß blocker-based regimens (OR 0.63, 95% CI 0.55 to 0.73 versus placebo compared to a non-significant 8% reduction in the odds on ACEI-based therapy). In the PROGRESS trial,[21] treatment with either perindopril or a combination of perindopril and indapamide led to a 26% RRR (95% CI 16 to 34%) in major vascular event rate and a 28% RRR (95% CI 17 to 38%) in risk of recurrent stroke compared to placebo. Most of this benefit was explained by those on combination therapy who had the biggest blood pressure reduction. Benefits were similar regardless of history of hypertension (Table 6.4).

Antihypertensive therapy is therefore recommended to both reduce risk of first and recurrent stroke and risk of other vascular events following ischaemic stroke, TIA, and intra-parenchymal haemorrhage. Therapy should be considered in all, although target blood pressure levels are not well defined. Data support the use of a combination of diuretic and ACE inhibitor therapies in the secondary prevention setting.

Diabetes

There is some suggestion that those with type 2 diabetes not requiring insulin who have suffered stroke be commenced on pioglitazone therapy. This is based only on subgroup analysis from the PROactive trial,[22] where a reduction in both fatal and non-fatal stroke was seen (Table 6.4).

All those with a diagnosis of stroke should be screened for the presence of diabetes mellitus and treated accordingly.

Cardioembolic stroke/atrial fibrillation

Presence of atrial fibrillation increased risk of both first stroke and recurrent stroke, and those with concurrent increased age, diabetes, congestive cardiac failure, previous stroke, and hypertension are at the highest risk. Scoring algorithms are now commonly employed to help predict stroke risk and identify those with atrial fibrillation most likely to benefit from anticoagulant treatment. An example is the

CHADS2 score, where the variables of presence of recent congestive cardiac failure, hypertension, age > 75 years, and diabetes mellitus are assigned one point and history of stroke or TIA two points. Those with a score of two or more (assuming no treatment) have a stroke risk of approximately 4% per annum, rising to 8.5% per annum in those with a score of four.

The most widely used and studied anticoagulant is warfarin, which inhibits synthesis of vitamin K-dependent clotting factors. In the primary prevention setting, warfarin treatment gives a hugely beneficial relative risk reduction of 68% for ischaemic stroke compared to placebo. In absolute terms, meta-analysis data showed the stroke rate fell from 4.5% per annum to 1.4% with warfarin treatment.[23] The recommended INR range is two to three. Aspirin also provides benefit but is clearly the inferior strategy.

Warfarin is similarly effective in the secondary preventative setting, giving a 40% reduction in the risk of major vascular events or death in those with atrial fibrillation and previous stroke. The timescale of initiation of anticoagulation in this setting is unclear. For example, in the European Atrial Fibrillation Trial,[24] nearly one-half of patients commenced anticoagulation within 14 days, although their neurological deficits were minor (Table 6.4). Thus, it is generally recommended that anticoagulation should be initiated within two weeks in those with AF and stroke and guidelines suggest the decision regarding timing be individualised. In those with large infarct volume and major clinical deficit, caution is probably justified, although in those with minor disability, anticoagulation is often started early. Regarding safety and risk of haemorrhage, warfarin can be considered safe in comparison to aspirin, with a major bleeding rate of 1.3% compared to 1% on aspirin or placebo.

Dual antiplatelet therapy with aspirin and clopidogrel has been compared to warfarin and offers inferior stroke protection at the cost of a similar burden of bleeding complications. In those deemed unsuitable for warfarin therapy, clopidogrel and aspirin may lead to fewer vascular events than aspirin alone, although the risk of major haemorrhage is also increased. The use of this strategy is not clear as yet.

There are a number of newer anticoagulant agents in development. One, dabigatran etexilate, has shown promise. In the RELY study,[25] dabigatran at a dose of 150 mg per day gave slightly lower risk of ischaemic stroke with similar risk of major haemorrhage. The main potential benefits of such new anticoagulants are not efficacy but a lack of requirement for dose adjustment and regular monitoring.

Anticoagulation with warfarin is the treatment of choice for prevention of recurrent stroke in those with cardioembolic stroke and for primary prevention in those with atrial fibrillation whose risk of stroke exceeds the likely risk of haemorrhage. In those deemed unsuitable for anticoagulation, aspirin is effective and therapy with aspirin and clopidogrel leads to fewer strokes but at the cost of increased haemorrhage risk.

Carotid artery intervention

Approximately 10–15% of ischaemic strokes are thought to be due to large artery atherosclerosis, most of which are associated with a stenosis of the ipsilateral extra-cranial carotid artery. This stenosis can be remedied by carotid endarterectomy (CEA) or by percutaneous placement of a carotid stent (Table 6.5).

Large randomized controlled trials found carotid endarterectomy to be superior to medical therapy in those who have symptomatic severe carotid stenosis. A pooled analysis of the major symptomatic stenosis trials[26] showed, in those with symptomatic severe ($\geq$ 70%) stenosis, surgery afforded a 15.6% absolute risk reduction (ARR) over five years and a smaller 4.5% ARR (p = 0.04) in those with moderate (50–69%) stenosis. Surgery slightly increased risk (by 2.2%) of stroke in those with less than 30% stenosis, but no effect on risk was seen in those with 30–49% stenosis or in the presence of near occlusion.

It is now known that early surgery, despite its inherent increased risk, is associated with greater absolute and relative risk reduction than delayed surgery. The difference is not small; in those with severe stenosis, surgery in those who were randomized to treatment within two weeks of symptoms afforded an ARR of 23% (95% CI 13.6 to 32.4%) compared to only 7.4% (95% CI –3.3 to 18.1%) if randomized after 12 weeks. Those with moderate stenosis also derived significant benefit if randomized within two weeks of their event. Thus, if treated early, those with a symptomatic 50–69% stenosis do derive benefit; this is greatest in men, those aged over 75, those with evidence of infarction, and those with hemispheric (rather than retinal) symptoms.

Peri-procedural risk is a key factor in determining benefit from carotid endarterectomy; the lower the absolute benefit from carotid endarterectomy (such as in younger female patients or asymptomatic disease), the lower the surgical complication rate requires to be to ensure benefit. It is generally accepted that this must be < 6% for those with severe stenosis but < 3% in those with moderate stenosis and with asymptomatic disease.

Carotid artery stenting (CAS) is a further treatment option and has not yet been proven to be superior, or perhaps not even equivalent to carotid endarterectomy. Results of individual trials have differed, perhaps due to differences peri-procedural complications rates and operator experience, sometimes in favor of endarterectomy and other times not. There are several important trials to consider.

The EVA -3S trial[27] included patients with at least 60% carotid stenosis and ipsilateral stroke within 120 days. It was terminated prematurely after inclusion of 527 patients; the 30-day incidence of stroke or death was 3.9% following carotid endarterectomy and 9.6% after stenting (RR 2.5, 95% CI 1.2 to 5.1). A further recent trial also failed to prove non-inferiority of carotid stenting. The SPACE trial[28] included 1200 patients with severe symptomatic (within six months) carotid stenosis. The rate of death or ipsilateral ischaemic stroke within 30 days was 6.84%

following stenting and 6.34% following endarterectomy (OR 1.09, 95% CI 0.69 to 1.72). In SPACE, interventional radiologists were required to show greater levels of experience than in EVA-3S before being included in the study. The CAVATAS trial[29] enrolled 504 patients with symptomatic carotid disease and compared CEA with carotid angioplasty (only one-fourth of patients received stents). The trial

TABLE 6.5 Clinical trials of carotid endarterectomy and carotid stenting for the prevention of stroke

Trial	Population	Primary endpoint	Intervention and primary endpoint rate
Pooled meta-analysis *N = 6000	Symptomatic stenosis	Any stroke or operative death	Absolute risk reduction for event following CEA 15.6%*. Relative risk reduction following CEA 0.5, 96% CI 0.4 to 0.6.
WALLSTENT N = 219	Symptomatic stenosis	Peri-procedural stroke rate	CAS 12.1% CEA 4.5% (p = 0.049)
EVA-3S N = 527	Symptomatic stenosis (> 60%)	Stroke or death within 30 days	CAS–9.6% CEA–3.9% Relative risk of event with CAS versus CEA 2.5, 95% CI 1.2 to 5.1.
SAPPHIRE N = 334	Symptomatic (> 50%) or asymptomatic (> 80%) stenosis	Death, stroke, or MI within 30 days or death or ipsilateral stroke from to one year	CAS 12.2% CEA 20.1% Absolute difference in event rate 7.9 %, 95% CI, –16.4 to 0.7
SPACE N = 1214	Symptomatic stenosis	Ipsilateral ischaemic stroke or death to 30 days after the procedure	CAS–9.8% CEA–7.8% Hazard ratio for event with CAS 1.1, 95% CI 0.75 to 1.61%
CREST N = 2502	Symptomatic or asymptomatic stenosis	Periprocedural stroke, MI, or death or ipsilateral stroke within four years	CAS 7.2% CEA 6.8% Hazard ratio for event with CAS 1.11, 95% CI 0.81 to 1.51
ICSS N = 1713	Symptomatic carotid artery stenosis	120-day rate of stroke, death, or procedural MI	CAS 8.5% CEA 5.2% Hazard ratio for event with CAS 1.69, 95% CI 1.16–2.45
ACST N=3120	Asymptomatic carotid stenosis (> 60%)	Five years risk of stroke or death	Immediate CEA–6.4% Indefinite deferral of CEA -11.8% Absolute difference in event rate following CEA 5.4%, 95% CI 3 to 7.8

* Figure is for > 70% stenosis. CEA = carotid endarterectomy, CAS = carotid artery stenosis, MI = myocardial infarction. Abbreviated trial names are given and full references are found at the end of the chapter.

also included participants with vertebrobasilar stenotic disease. The 30-day risk of stroke or death was similar (9.9% with CEA and 10% with CAS) with no difference in recurrent stroke rate at one year. The peri-surgical risk was however higher than that suggested as the maximum accepted level in consensus guidelines. In the SAPPHIRE trial,[30] 334 patients deemed at high risk during CEA were randomized to either CEA or CAS with emboli detection. Patients either had at least 50% symptomatic stenosis or asymptomatic 80% stenosis. The endpoint was a composite of death, stroke, or MI within 30 days after the event or ipsilateral stroke between 31 days and one year. This was less frequent following stenting (12.2% versus 20.1%, absolute difference of 7.9%, 95% CI –0.7 to 16.4%) and the non-inferiority criteria were met (p = 0.004 for non-inferiority). The benefit was largely driven by a reduction in MI in those treated with CAS. Importantly, the peri-procedural rate of stroke, MI, or death following CAS was only 4.8% in this study, in comparison to the higher rates in other trials, and the peri-procedural complication rate following endarterectomy was high at 9.9%. The recent Carotid Revascularization Endarterectomy versus Stenting Trial (CREST)[31] showed stenting to be similar in terms of a combined endpoint, which included MI, stroke, and vascular death but higher risk of stroke at 30 days. Younger patients (< 70 years) appeared to do better with stenting. It is worth noting that nearly half of the patients included in CREST were asymptomatic and that peri-procedural stroke rates were low with both treatments.

Carotid endarterectomy in the primary prevention setting (those with asymptomatic stenosis) has also been the subject of large randomized controlled trials. In general, these trials support benefit in those with at least moderate stenosis, although the absolute benefit appears small and thus mandates a low peri-procedural complication rate to give benefit. For example, in the most recent trial, the Asymptomatic Carotid Surgery Trial,[33] 3120 patients were randomized to either immediate endarterectomy or indefinite deferral of endarterectomy. The peri-operative rate of stroke or death was 3.1% following CEA. Even when these events were considered, the five-year risk of stroke or death was lower following CEA (6.4% versus 11.8%, ARR 5.4%, 95% CI 3 to 7.8) but on subgroup analysis, benefit was not apparent in those aged over 75 years.

BEHAVIOURAL RISK FACTORS
Smoking cessation
There are no randomised controlled trials to evaluate the efficacy of smoking cessation therapy after stroke. However, it is generally regarded as an important strategy given compelling data from observational studies and the other health benefits associated with stopping. Observational data suggest that stopping smoking affords a reduction in stroke risk and that risk returns to that of a non-smoker after five years.

Excess alcohol intake

The relationship between alcohol intake and stroke risk is complex, unproven, and somewhat controversial. It is generally accepted that the relationship is J-shaped with heavy drinkers having an increased risk and likewise those who consume no alcohol.

Guidelines suggest that those who are heavy drinkers should be advised to eliminate or reduce their consumption of alcohol.

Weight reduction/physical exercise

As yet, no data exist to suggest benefit from weight reduction in obese individuals with stroke, but given the benefits on metabolic parameters such as lipid levels and blood pressure, guidelines suggest weight management is encouraged through lifestyle measures.

SUMMARY

There are thus a number of effective preventative therapies for both the primary and secondary prevention of stroke. Strategies include antiplatelet therapy and lipid-lowering therapy to prevent ischaemic stroke, anticoagulant therapy to prevent cardioembolic ischaemic stroke and blood pressure reduction, treatment of prevalent diabetes, lifestyle therapy, and behavioural modification to prevent all stroke subtypes.

REFERENCES

1. Asplund K, Berman P, Blomstrand C, *et al.* How do stroke units improve patient outcomes? A collaborative systematic review of the randomized trials. *Stroke.* 1997; **28**: 2139–44.
2. Leonardi-Bee J, Bath PMW, Phillips SJ, *et al.* Blood pressure and clinical outcomes in the international stroke trial. *Stroke.* 2002; **33**: 1315–20.
3. Sandset EC, Bath PMW, Boysen G, *et al.* The angiotensin-receptor blocker candesartan for treatment of acute stroke (SCAST): a randomised, placebo-controlled, double-blind trial. *Lancet.* 2011; **377**: 741–50.
4. Gray CS, Hildreth AJ, Sandercock PA, *et al.* Glucose-potassium-insulin infusions in the management of post-stroke hyperglycaemia: the UK Glucose Insulin in Stroke Trial (GIST-UK). *Lancet Neurology.* 2007; **6**: 397–406.
5. Hacke W, Kaste M, Bluhmki E, *et al.* Thrombolysis with alteplase 3 to 4.5 hours after acute ischemic stroke. *NEJM.* 2008; **359**: 1317–29.
6. Hacke W, Donnan G, Fieschi C, *et al.* Association of outcome with early stroke treatment: pooled analysis of ATLANTIS, ECASS, and NINDS rt-PA stroke trials. *Lancet.* 2004; **363**: 768–74.
7. Wahlgren N, Ahmed N, Davalos A, *et al.* Thrombolysis with alteplase for acute ischaemic stroke in the Safe Implementation of Thrombolysis in Stroke-Monitoring Study (SITS-MOST): an observational study. *Lancet.* 2007; **369**: 275–82.

8. Furlan A, Higashida R, Wechsler L, *et al.* Intra-arterial prourokinase for acute ischemic stroke. The PROACT II study: a randomized controlled trial. Prolyse in acute cerebral thromboembolism. *JAMA.* 1999; **282**: 2003-11.

9. Vahedi K, Hofmeijer J, Juettler E, *et al.* Early decompressive surgery in malignant infarction of the middle cerebral artery: a pooled analysis of three randomised controlled trials. *Lancet Neurology.* 2007; **6**: 215-22.

10. Antiplatelet Trialists' Collaboration. Collaborative meta-analysis of randomised trials of antiplatelet therapy for prevention of death, myocardial infarction, and stroke in high-risk patients: *BMJ.* 2002; **324**: 71-86.

11. CAPRIE Steering Committee. A randomised, blinded, trial of clopidogrel versus aspirin in patients at risk of ischaemic events (CAPRIE). *Lancet.* 1996; **348**: 1329-39.

12. Halkes PH, van Gijn J, Kappelle LJ, *et al.* Aspirin plus dipyridamole versus aspirin alone after cerebral ischaemia of arterial origin (ESPRIT): randomised controlled trial. *Lancet.* 2006; **367**: 1665-73.

13. Bhatt DL, Fox KA, Hacke W, *et al.* Clopidogrel and aspirin versus aspirin alone for the prevention of atherothrombotic events. *NEJM.* 2006; **354**: 1706-17.

14. Diener HC, Bogousslavsky J, Brass LM, *et al.* Aspirin and clopidogrel compared with clopidogrel alone after recent ischaemic stroke or transient ischaemic attack in high-risk patients (MATCH): randomised, double-blind, placebo-controlled trial. *Lancet.* 2004; **364**: 331-7.

15. Markus HS, Droste DW, Kaps M, *et al.* Dual antiplatelet therapy with clopidogrel and aspirin in symptomatic carotid stenosis evaluated using Doppler embolic signal detection: the Clopidogrel and Aspirin for Reduction of Emboli in Symptomatic Carotid Stenosis (CARESS) trial. *Circulation.* 2005; **111**: 2233-40.

16. Sacco RL, Diener HC, Yusuf S, *et al.* Aspirin and extended-release dipyridamole versus clopidogrel for recurrent stroke. *NEJM.* 2008; **359**: 1238-51.

17. Larosa JC, He J, Vupputuri S. Effect of statins on risk of coronary disease: A meta-analysis of randomized controlled trials. *JAMA.* 1999; **282**: 2340-6.

18. Collins R, Armitage J, Parish S, *et al.* MRC/BHF Heart Protection Study of cholesterol lowering with simvastatin in 20536 high-risk individuals: a randomised placebo-controlled trial. *Lancet.* 2002; **360**: 7-22.

19. Amarenco P, Bogousslavsky J, Callahan A, *et al.* High-dose atorvastatin after stroke or transient ischemic attack. *NEJM.* 2006; **355**: 549-59.

20. Zhang H, Thijs L, Staessen JA. Blood pressure lowering for primary and secondary prevention of stroke. *Hypertension.* 2006; **48**: 187-95.

21. The PROGRESS Study Group. A trial of a perindopril-based blood-pressure-lowering regimen among 6105 individuals with previous stroke or transient ischaemic attack. *Lancet.* 2001; **358**: 1033-41.

22. Dormandy JA, Charbonnel B, Eckland DJA, *et al.* Secondary prevention of macrovascular events in patients with type 2 diabetes in the PROactive Study (PROspective pioglitazone clinical trial in macrovascular events): a randomised controlled trial. *Lancet.* 2005; **366**: 1279-89.

23. Laupacis A, Boysen G, Connolly S, *et al.* Risk-factors for stroke and efficacy of antithrombotic therapy in atrial-fibrillation: analysis of pooled data from 5 randomized controlled trials. *Archives of Internal Medicine.* 1994; **154**: 1449-57.

24. Koudstaal PJ, Dehaene I, Dhooghe M, *et al.* Secondary prevention in nonrheumatic atrial-fibrillation after transient ischemic attack or minor stroke. *Lancet.* 1993; **342**: 1255–62.
25. Connolly SJ, Ezekowitz MD, Yusuf S. Dabigatran versus warfarin in patients with atrial fibrillation. *NEJM.* 2009; **361**: 1139–51.
26. Rothwell PM, Eliasziw M, Gutnikov SA, *et al.* Analysis of pooled data from the randomised controlled trials of endarterectomy for symptomatic carotid stenosis. *Lancet.* 2003; **361**: 107–16.
27. Mas J, Chatellier G, Beyssen B, *et al.* Endarterectomy versus stenting in patients with symptomatic severe carotid stenosis. *NEJM.* 2006; **355**: 1660–71.
28. Ringleb PA, Allenberg J, Berger J. 30-day results from the SPACE trial of stent-protected angioplasty versus carotid endarterectomy in symptomatic patients: a randomised non-inferiority trial. *Lancet.* 2006; **368**: 1239–47.
29. Brown MM, Rogers J, Bland JM. Endovascular versus surgical treatment in patients with carotid stenosis in the Carotid and Vertebral Artery Transluminal Angioplasty Study (CAVATAS): a randomised trial. *Lancet.* 2001; **357**: 1729–37.
30. Yadav JS, Wholey MH, Kuntz RE, *et al.* Protected carotid-artery stenting versus endarterectomy in high-risk patients. *NEJM.* 2004; **351**: 1493–501.
31. Brott TG, Hobson RW, Howard PH. Stenting versus endarterectomy for treatment of carotid-artery stenosis (CREST). *NEJM.* 2010; **363**: 11–23.
32. Alberts MJ. Results of a multicenter prospective randomized trial of carotid artery stenting vs. carotid endarterectomy. *Stroke.* 2001; **32**: 325.
33. Halliday A, Mansfield A, Marro J, *et al.* Prevention of disabling and fatal strokes by successful carotid endarterectomy in patients without recent neurological symptoms: randomised controlled trial. *Lancet.* 2004; **363**: 1491–502.

CHAPTER 7

Transient ischaemic attacks

OUTLINE

Transient ischemic attacks (TIAs) are brief episodes of neurological dysfunction that arise as a consequence of focal ischaemia but are not associated with cerebral infarction. In recent years, they have been the subject of intensive study, leading to a reevaluation of their definition, prognostic significance, and management. This chapter will provide an overview of the clinical significance, epidemiology, evaluation, and treatment of patients with TIA.

DEFINITION

The precise definition of transient ischaemic attack is changing. It has historically been defined as a focal neurological deficit of sudden onset and presumed vascular origin lasting up to 24 hours. When this definition was agreed, approximately 40 years ago, the arbitrary 24-hour time limit was included to differentiate TIA from stroke, as it was assumed that the short-lived symptoms would not be associated with any permanent damage to the brain. Subsequent advances in brain imaging have revealed evidence of new cerebral infarction in patients with symptoms of less than 24 hours' duration. This finding has prompted a re-evaluation of the definition of TIA, with a move away from an arbitrary temporal threshold towards a tissue-based definition that is more reliant upon brain imaging. As such, the revised definition of TIA as a 'brief episode of neurological dysfunction caused by focal brain or retinal ischemia, with clinical symptoms typically lasting less than one hour, and without evidence of acute infarction' has been widely adopted.

PATHOPHYSIOLOGICAL CONSIDERATIONS AND EPIDEMIOLOGY

Because of their brief duration, the mechanistic basis of transient ischemic attacks is difficult to study. It is generally assumed that the pathophysiological processes which cause TIA are similar to those that cause ischaemic stroke (as discussed earlier). TIAs may have a haemodynamic basis in the context of significant extra-cranial or intracranial arterial stenosis, which may be provoked or compounded by transient reduction in blood pressure. They may be caused by embolism from the heart or from proximal arteries, or from small vessel lipohyalinosis involving small penetrating vessels arising from larger intracranial arteries. More rarely, TIAs have been associated with haematological disorders such as severe anaemia, polycythemia, or other hyperviscosity states.

Calculating the incidence and prevalence of TIA is also a challenge, as due to their brief and self-limiting nature, they may not be recognised or appropriately recorded by the patient or doctor. It is therefore likely that many epidemiological studies underestimate the true number of TIAs in the community. Probably the most reliable data come from very carefully conducted community-based studies such as the Oxford Vascular study, which reported an incidence rate for TIA across a whole population of 0.66 per 1000 patients per year. As with stroke, the incidence of TIA increases very sharply with age, reaching > 6 per 1000 patients per year in those over 85 years.

PROGNOSTIC SIGNIFICANCE

TIA has long been identified as a strong marker of vascular risk. Up to 40% of patients presenting with stroke give a history consistent with prior TIA, the majority occurring in the days or weeks before the stroke occurred. Prompt identification, risk stratification, and treatment of patients presenting with TIA is therefore advantageous. In recent years, a number of studies have sought to identify which TIA patients are at particularly high risk of stroke. Use of a simple risk stratification score (the ABCD2 score) has been shown to predict short-term risk of stroke in TIA patients using easily measured clinical parameters. Patients presenting with TIA score points for each of the following factors:

- age 60 years or more (1 point)
- blood pressure on first measurement 140/90 mm Hg or more (1 point)
- focal weakness (2 points) or speech impairment without weakness (1 point)
- duration 60 minutes (2 points) or 10 to 59 minutes (1 point)
- diabetes (1 point)

Early risk of stroke (within two days of TIA) approximates to 0% for scores of 0 or 1, 1.3% for 2 or 3, 4.1% for 4 or 5, and 8.1% for scores of 6 or 7. The ABCD2 score is therefore a simple risk stratification instrument that has been validated in a number of cohorts. It uses readily available clinical information and can be applied in primary care. More complex risk stratification is possible following TIA with the incorporation of imaging findings: for example, patients with transient symptoms but a new infarct on brain imaging (in other words, patients who would be classified as 'stroke' under the new taxonomy) or with significant carotid stenosis (*see* below) are at significantly higher risk than those with no new infarct or stenosis.

INVESTIGATION OF THE PATIENT WITH SUSPECTED TIA

The high risk of stroke after TIA mandates prompt evaluation of all patients suspected to have neurovascular symptoms. Imaging is a key component of the evaluation of patients with suspected TIA. The goal is to demonstrate a vascular basis for the symptoms, to gain an insight into the aetiology of an event (through identification of a potential cause such as stenosis of large arteries or visualisation of a cardiac source of emboli), and to exclude certain stroke mimics such as intracranial space-occupying lesions.

Brain imaging

Choice of brain imaging modality is frequently driven by availability. In the UK, computed tomography (CT) of brain is the most readily accessible technique. The diagnostic yield of CT is relatively low following transient neurological symptoms, with evidence of cerebral infarction (new or established) in less than 20%, and evidence of a non-vascular pathology in less than 5%. Magnetic resonance imaging more expensive and less accessible; however, when performed early, it provides a greater diagnostic yield, with a lesion visible on diffusion-weighted MRI in approximately 40% of patients.

Vessel imaging

Patients with TIA in carotid artery territory should undergo imaging of the extracranial carotid arteries as swiftly as feasible. The most widely used modality is ultrasound, which provides a well-tolerated and non-invasive assessment of the carotid bifurcation and much of the extracranial internal carotid artery. Ultrasound imaging of patients with TIA or minor stroke will detect 50% or greater stenosis on an internal carotid artery in between 8% and 31% of this group.

Magnetic resonance angiography (MRA) and computed tomographic angiography (CTA) are alternatives to ultrasound techniques. These modalities are less readily available and generally less well-tolerated (or in some cases impossible, such as MR imaging in those with permanent pacemaker units or severe claustrophobia) but allow imaging of a larger portion of the vascular tree as vessels between the aortic arch and Circle of Willis can be visualised.

Despite many studies, no optimal strategy for vessel imaging has emerged, and in most cases, the choice of strategy is driven by local availability. As a general rule, when the initial test suggests a stenosis and surgery is being considered, a second confirmatory test using a different modality should be employed prior to intervention.

Cardiac testing

Optimal cardiac investigation of TIA patients is difficult as there is a paucity of data to guide clinicians. Extensive cardiac work-up in those with a history of TIA or stroke but no history or examination findings consistent with cardiac disease is generally unrewarding, with fewer than 3% having evidence of a cardioembolic source on transthoracic echocardiography (TTE). Transoesophageal echocardiography (TOE) has a greater yield of cardiac abnormality (particularly atrial thrombi, atrial septal aneurysm, and aortic arch atheroma) but is an invasive technique that is usually reserved for patients in whom a cardioembolic source is strongly suspected. Prolonged cardiac monitoring may be of value in this group of patients, particularly if a history of palpitation is obtained. Monitoring for 24 hours is standard, but there is some evidence that more prolonged monitoring can provide greater yields, with a four-day monitor demonstrating paroxysmal atrial fibrillation in 14% of patients in whom 24-hour monitoring had shown no significant abnormality.

PREVENTION OF FURTHER VASCULAR EVENTS FOLLOWING TIA

A number of strategies can be used to reduce risk of stroke or other vascular events in patients with TIA. As the risk of subsequent stroke is known to be particularly high in the days following a TIA, swift initiation of secondary preventative treatment is the goal. The strategies used in patients with TIA are the same as those used for prevention of recurrent stroke: combination of antiplatelet therapy, statin, and antihypertensive treatment together with dietary and lifestyle advice where appropriate are the mainstay of treatment. In a selected group of patients at particularly elevated risk, additional strategies such as oral anticoagulation, carotid revascularisation, and improved diabetic control should be used. The benefit of these strategies is well established, and the major challenge facing clinicians is providing them very early after the onset of TIA. The potential benefit of a swift and aggressive paradigm for investigation and treatment is huge: in one study, an 80% reduction in 90-day stroke risk was reported after the institution of a fast-track clinic to assess and treat TIA patients. Ideally, the evaluation and treatment of these patients should be completed within hours of symptom onset. The high risk of early recurrent stroke and effectiveness of early preventative strategies make TIA a medical emergency.

CHAPTER 8

Stroke mimics

INTRODUCTION

There are a number of other conditions that may resemble stroke and confuse clinicians. In fact, significant proportions (up to 30%) of 'stroke' admissions have been found to be a stroke mimic, and ways to increase diagnostic accuracy have been the focus of much work.[1, 2, 3, 4] History is critical in identifying the disguised culprit as is clinical examination and neuroimaging. The latter does not always identify a definite lesion, and the diagnosis of stroke remains mainly clinical. The reliability of clinical diagnosis in stroke, on the other hand, has been found to be moderate.[5]

Here we discuss other clinical entities that must be considered. Exclusive or characteristic features are highlighted, as are instruments that may be helpful in making the correct diagnosis.

STROKE MIMICS

It can be argued that most of these entities warrant early neurological assessment by a stroke neurologist or stroke physician. This is in order to facilitate accurate diagnosis and thus either acute stroke therapy or rapidly address the underlying condition. Given their reasonably high incidence and the unpredictable pattern of emergency admissions, we would recommend that experienced physicians are involved at an early stage in the diagnostic process, ideally in the emergency department. Commonly encountered mimics are presented in Table 8.1.

Migraine

Migraine is among the most common causes of severe headache, has a predilection for women, and can easily be mistaken for stroke due to focal neurological deficits often associated with it, especially when aura is of acute onset or not associated with headache. Migraine can be subdivided to three clinical subtypes: (1) *classic migraine* or migraine associated with aura; this subtype has recently been postulated to be associated with increased risk of stroke;[6] (2) *common migraine* or migraine not

TABLE 8.1 Causes of presentations mimicking stroke

Migraine
Seizure
Syncope
Transient global amnesia
Vestibular dysfunction
Sepsis
Toxic-metabolic encephalopathy
Space-occupying lesion
Delirium
Dementia
Acute peripheral neuropathy
Spinal cord lesion
Multiple sclerosis
Functional/hysterical

associated with aura; and (3) *migraine variant* (comprising migrainous vertigo, retinal, hemiplegic, ophthalmoplegic, and basilar migraine). No aura implies no focal neurological deficits that may mimic stroke; thus, types (1) and (3) are of particular relevance to stroke.

Classic migraine

- The headache associated with nausea, photophobia, and phonophobia may be heralded by prodromal symptoms (appearing 24–48 hours prior). These may comprise such diverse symptoms as hyperactivity, euphoria, lethargy, depression, frequent yawning, and craving for certain foods.[7]
- Aura precedes the headache (usually by 1–2 hours) in the majority of cases. Classic visual findings are flashing lights and the pathognomonic fortification spectrum, which usually begins as a paracentral scotoma. Hemianopia or monocular blindness are sometimes seen but more rarely.
- Sensory symptoms comprise numbness, tingling, or even pain, usually affecting the hand, arm, and face. Unilateral paraesthesias and numbness often involve the extremities distally and may also be peri-oral.
- Unilateral motor weakness may affect the hand, arm, and face on the same side.[8]
- Dysphasia is uncommon but may be seen and Wernicke's dysphasia is a recognised feature.[9]
- Aura typically resolves within one hour, but in many, motor symptoms may persist for longer. An aura lasting longer than one hour is indicative of complicated migraine.

Migraine variants

- *Aura without headache* is a variant (also known as *migraine equivalent*) that may be confused with transient ischemic attacks, especially in older patients[10] and when it is of acute onset.

- *Migrainous vertigo* refers to episodic vertigo in patients with a history of migraine. It is essentially a vestibular disorder manifesting with positional vertigo or dizziness and relies on exclusion of other causes.[11] Isolated acute vertigo may be seen with brainstem ischaemia, although the latter is more commonly associated with other brainstem symptoms.
- *Retinal migraine* is an interesting but rare entity that may manifest as episodes of monocular scotomata or blindness associated with headache and usually resolving within an hour. Interestingly, onset may be acute[10] and recurrent episodes may lead to permanent visual loss.[12]
- *Hemiplegic migraine*, whether sporadic or familial, is associated with motor aura, during which transient hemiplegia is seen. Other aural symptoms accompany these episodes, most frequently sensory, visual, and dysphasic. Basilar features are seen in more than two-thirds of cases, and severe attacks may precipitate prolonged hemiparesis, confusion, coma, fever, seizures, and permanent cerebellar signs (such as nystagmus, ataxia, and dysarthria).[13]
- *Ophthalmoplegic migraine*, according to the International Headache Society, is repeated attacks of headache with migrainous characteristics associated with paresis of one or more ocular cranial nerves (most commonly the oculomotor) in the absence of any demonstrable intracranial lesion. The paresis typically occurs at the height of an attack of a unilateral cephalgia, which primarily localises in the orbital region. The paresis may persist for weeks despite resolution of the cephalgia, and recovery is gradual. The attacks commonly affect children, may be atypical, featuring long-lasting headache, and recurrent attacks may progressively precipitate nerve damage and thus incomplete recovery.[14]
- Aura is not usually a feature of *basilar migraine* but brainstem signs are the predominant feature. Dizziness, vertigo, dysarthria, diplopia, impaired hearing and tinnitus, ataxia, bilateral paresthesias, and altered consciousness may be seen. All these features may accompany familial hemiplegic migraine, but motor weakness should not be seen in basilar migraine.[15] This variant was first described by Bickerstaff in 1961 as a rare syndrome affecting young women.[16] The term 'Bickerstaff's migraine' is nowadays reserved for extreme forms of basilar migraine, involving total blindness in addition to the above brainstem findings, while loss of consciousness and a confusional state is seen in a proportion. These symptoms may last for 20–30 minutes but altered perception sometimes persists for up to five days.[8]

Is it migraine or stroke?

- Clinical examination may be unhelpful in distinguishing migraine from stroke (when symptoms persist) or transient ischaemic attack (when symptoms resolve), although one may be more suspecting of migraine in a young individual with no vascular risk factors, but this alone should not exclude stroke.

- History is more crucial than examination here, as a past personal or family occurrence of migraine attacks is a strong pointer to migraine versus stroke.
- Prodromal symptoms are suggestive of migraine, as is a rapid but not sudden onset. The migrainous aura usually spreads and maximises over 10–15 minutes, whether TIA and stroke are of abrupt, sudden onset, at which point symptoms are at their maximum. The situation is made more complex when the aura is of sudden onset and when the migraine is the headache-free variant.

Seizure
Definitions and classification

Seizure is defined as the clinical manifestation of abnormally excessive brain neuron discharge. Epilepsy on the other hand is defined as recurrent seizures in the absence of an identifiable underlying cause.[17]

The classification of epilepsy is complex, and the scheme recently proposed by the International League Against Epilepsy (ILAE) is briefly presented in Table 8.2. We recommend thinking of and subdividing epilepsy into three broad categories:[18]

- *generalised epilepsies*: associated with diffuse hyperexcitability of membranes and involving loss of consciousness
- *focal epilepsies*: caused by a focus of cortical neuronal discharge, which might spread and thus manifest as focal neurological deficit evolving to more global signs
- *provoked seizures*: secondary to an immediate underlying cause (*see* below).

Causes

An underlying aetiology is only found in approximately one-third of patients presenting with seizure in late life. Pathologies that may present with seizure that may be encountered in clinical practice comprise trauma; acute alcohol excess or withdrawal from chronic consumption; tumour; metabolic disturbances; infection; multiple sclerosis; cerebral degeneration; drugs that lower the epileptic threshold in predisposed individuals (e.g., tricyclic antidepressants, isoniazid, antihistamines, quinolones, and alcohol) or non-compliance with prescribed therapy; and, interestingly, cerebrovascular disease. In fact, the prevalence of epilepsy after stroke is thought to be 6–15%, and recurrent stroke may well be confused as seizure.

Clinical manifestations

Seizure symptoms can be thought of as focal and generalised:

- *focal symptoms include*: focal limb jerking; focal paraesthesia; olfactory, gustatory, and visual hallucinations; and swallowing and chewing movements
- *generalised symptoms comprise*: generalised stiffening (tonic); repeated generalised jerking (clonic); intermittent symmetrical jerking (myotonic); absence with no focal symptoms; and atonic drop attacks.

TABLE 8.2 Classification of epilepsy

I *Partial (focal, local) seizures*
A Simple partial seizures (consciousness not impaired)
1 With motor symptoms
2 With somatosensory or special sensory symptoms
3 With autonomic symptoms
4 With psychic symptoms
B Complex partial seizures (with impairment of consciousness)
1 Beginning as simple partial seizures and progressing to impairment of consciousness
(a) With no other features
(b) With features as in simple partial seizures
(c) With automatisms
2 With impairment of consciousness at onset
(a) With no other features
(b) With features as in simple partial seizures
(c) With automatisms
C Partial seizures evolving to secondarily generalized seizures
1 Simple partial seizures evolving to generalized seizures
2 Complex partial seizures evolving to generalized seizures
3 Simple partial seizures evolving to complex partial seizures to generalized seizures
II *Generalized seizures (convulsive or non-convulsive)*
A 1 Absence seizures
2 Atypical absence seizures
B Myoclonic seizures
C Clonic seizures
D Tonic seizures
E Tonic-clonic seizures
F Atonic seizures (astatic seizures)
III *Unclassified epileptic seizures*

Of more interest to stroke are the post-ictal transient focal neurological deficits. Todd used the term 'epileptic hemiplegia' in his 1854 description[19] and the syndrome is often referred to as post-epileptic paralysis. Post-epileptic symptoms are variable and comprise hemiparesis, hemianopia, monocular blindness, pupillary dilatation, gaze palsies, dysphasia, and confusion, all of which may last from half an hour to 36 hours, with a mean of 15 hours.[20]

It comes as no surprise that transient brain ischaemia underlies the above stroke-like postictal manifestations of seizure: perfusion MRI studies have recently demonstrated reversible hemispheric hypoperfusion with accompanying transient but marked cerebrovascular dysfunction during the postictal phase.[21]

Is it seizure or stroke?

- Misdiagnosing seizure as transient ischaemic attack should be avoided by thorough assessment. However, carotid disease may occasionally present with limb jerking or twitching that lasts for seconds and is coarse and more pronounced distally. Such attacks may be accompanied by motor weakness or dysphasia and may very occasionally be mistaken for seizures,[17] but careful evaluation and a thorough clinical history should prevent this from occurring.

- The neurological deficits that can follow seizure can easily be confused with acute stroke. Even neuroimaging in such a context may be unhelpful by revealing pronounced hypoperfusion, pointing to evolving stroke. An accurate medical history would easily allow accurate diagnosis.

- Electroencephalography (EEG) is essential in the evaluation for seizure but has a sensitivity of only 20–55%.[22-25] Interictal epileptiform discharges may also be seen in healthy subjects with no history of epilepsy. This proportion has been found to be 2.2%[26] but may be slightly higher in adults with neurological or psychiatric pathologies.[27] To confuse matters further, focal slowing is a feature seen on the electroencephalogram of stroke patients.[28] In other words, EEG is useful but not diagnostic, and the diagnosis of epilepsy should be left to expert hands.

- It should be emphasised that seizure and stroke are not mutually exclusive and, indeed, the frequent occurrence of epileptic seizure at the onset of a cerebrovascular accident, more commonly haemorrhagic, is well established.[29-31]

Syncope
Definitions

The European Society of Cardiology defines syncope as *'A transient self-limited loss of consciousness, usually leading to falling. The onset is relatively rapid, and the subsequent recovery is spontaneous, complete, and relatively prompt. The underlying mechanism is a transient global cerebral hypoperfusion'*.[32] It is important that syncope is distinguished from dizziness, presyncope, vertigo, and drop attacks, none of which lead to loss of consciousness.[33]

Causes of syncope

Neural causes comprise vasovagal attacks (the most common culprit), situational syncope, and carotid sinus syncope. Cardiac syncope can be either due to structural heart disease or dysrrhythmia (second most common). Other causes include orthostatic hypotension, psychiatric illness, medications, and neurological disease, while a clear aetiology is never elucidated in approximately one-third of cases.[33]

Is it syncope or stroke?

- Brainstem ischaemia with impairment of the ascending reticular activating system and bihemispheric dysfunction would be responsible for loss of consciousness. However, syncope is by definition a transient, self-limited event, and in the absence of other neurological deficits, syncope from cerebrovascular disease is thought to be rare.[34]

- Transient vertebrobasilar insufficiency, a form of TIA, can lead to syncope and vertigo, ataxia, and sensory deficits may be seen.[34]

- In the same manner as seizure, syncope and TIA are not mutually exclusive. An accurate history exploring symptoms of brainstem dysfunction and any focal neurology present at the time of attack (if not resolved by the time of medical attention) would be invaluable.[35]

Transient global amnesia
What is it?

Transient global amnesia is an interesting clinical entity characterised by sudden onset anterograde amnesia (inability to form new memories), often associated with retrograde amnesia that may last for 24 hours. It has an incidence of three to eight per 100 000 and tends to affect patients from 50 to 70 years of age.[36]

A series of recent imaging studies has demonstrated hyperintense lesions in the hippocampal formation, and the vulnerability of hippocampal (CA1) neurons to metabolic stress has been implicated in the postulated pathobiology of the impaired memory circuits.[36]

Relevance to stroke

Transient global amnesia (TGA) is occasionally confused with stroke or transient ischaemic attack. Important points to note are the following.

- Stroke and TIA may be associated with temporary memory impairment as accompanying features of other focal neurology. The absence of other neurological symptoms or signs with the amnesia suggests TGA.
- The typical TGA patient tends to repeatedly ask questions about the present circumstances during the episode (which usually lasts no more than 24 hours). There is normally permanent memory loss from that short period.
- Most patients are middle-aged or elderly people and present with no other cognitive or focal neurological deficit.

TGA may mimic other pathologies, such as acute confusional state and complex partial seizure, and diagnostic criteria have been postulated[37] (summarised in Table 8.3).

TABLE 8.3 Diagnostic criteria of transient global amnesia

- Attack must be witnessed
- Acute onset of anterograde amnesia must be present
- No alteration in consciousness must be present
- No cognitive impairment other than amnesia must be present
- No loss of personal identity must be present
- No focal neurology or epileptic features must be present
- No recent history of head trauma or seizures must be present
- Attack must resolve within 24 hours
- Other causes of amnesia must be excluded

Non-stroke vestibulopathy
Overview

Vertere in Latin means *to turn*, and *verto* is *spinning*. Vertigo can be defined as hallucination of movement, an abnormal perception of movement of the patient or their surroundings that may or may not be rotational.

Motion is sensed by the vestibular system, which comprises the semicircular canals and the otolith organs. Signals are relayed from each of the right and left vestibular labyrinths to the central nervous system via the vestibular portion of CN VIII, to the vestibular nuclei in the brainstem, and subsequently to the cerebellum, ocular motor nuclei, and spinal cord, with more complex projections to the cerebrum. The cerebellum coordinates this orchestra of signals and interconnections, with a role in modulating vestibulo-ocular and vestibule-spinal pathways. These play a role in coordinating motion with eye movement and posture coordination, respectively. The relayed signals are compared centrally. Any differences are perceived as motion and a unilateral vestibulopathy, which would naturally impair signal transmission on the affected side, will be misinterpreted by the central nervous system as motion (hallucination of motion or vertigo).[38]

A deficit at any level in the above circuit, whether at the vestibule-labyrinthine apparatus, CN VIII, brainstem vestibular nuclei, or cerebellum, may lead to the illusion of movement of vertigo. Vertigo of sudden or vague new onset is a common presenting complaint in medical assessment units. Diagnosis can be challenging, and the presence of cerebellar symptoms may be alarming as to possible stroke as the culprit. It may thus be difficult to differentiate stroke from non-stroke vestibulopathy.

Causes of vertigo

These can be peripheral and central. Acute onset does not always imply cerebrovascular accident, as peripheral or non-stroke central aetiologies may present acutely. An overview of differential diagnoses is given in Table 8.4.

Non-stroke vestibulopathies

- Any of the above aetiologies may be mistaken for stroke but most bear certain features that would allow the experienced clinician to distinguish, mainly with the aid of the clinical history.
- Therefore, BPPV involves repeated and predictably provoked brief lasting attacks of periodic vertigo lacking other neurological signs. The Dix-Hallpike maneuver is positive in only 50 to 80% of patients with BPPV and a positive test would be supportive of the diagnosis.[39]
- Ménière's disease involves episodic vertigo typically associated with hearing loss, unilateral tinnitus, and ear fullness, and its diagnosis is suggested by the clinical history.

TABLE 8.4 Causes of vertigo

Peripheral
- Vestibular neuritis (also known as vestibular neuronitis, labyrinthitis, neurolabyrinthitis, and acute peripheral vestibulopathy)
- Benign paroxysmal positional vertigo (BPPV)
- Ramsay Hunt syndrome
- Ménière's disease
- Acoustic neuroma
- Aminoglycoside toxicity
- Otitis media

Central
- Brainstem ischaemia
- Cerebellar infarction and haemorrhage
- Migrainous vertigo
- Chiari malformation
- Multiple sclerosis
- Episodic ataxia type II

- Otoscopy would help identify the ear canal vesicles of Ramsay Hunt and the bulging tympanic membrane in otitis media. Aminoglycosides on the other hand tend to be peripherally vestibulotoxic but their effects are bilateral and vertigo is not a feature, although oscillopsia and disequilibrium are and, of course, a history of aminoglycoside use would give away the diagnosis.[40]
- Migrainous vertigo would involve migrainous headaches, at least occasionally, as part of this recurrent disease complex.
- The congenital Chiari I malformation, whereby the cerebellar tonsils extend below the foramen magnum, may be associated with gait instability, downbeat nystagmus, and vertigo. The diagnosis is easily confirmed with magnetic resonance imaging.
- Plaques involving the vestibular nerve may be associated with acute vertigo and other peripheral signs but other neurological deficits (such as pupillary afferent defect and long tract signs) would raise suspicion for demyelination. Of course, other causes, such as the more common BPPV, may be responsible for symptoms of vertigo in patients with established multiple sclerosis, and these should be considered.[41]
- Episodic ataxia type II is autosomal dominant and is characterised by recurrent episodes of vertigo, nystagmus, ataxia, nausea and vomiting since childhood or early adulthood life.[42] The lack of risk factors for cerebrovascular disease and a family history of vertigo attacks would be pointers to this rare diagnosis.

Stroke vestibulopathies

- Cerebellar strokes, whether infarction or haemorrhage, may cause vertigo, nausea, and vomiting in a presentation resembling acute peripheral vestibulopathy. Profound ataxia, impaired walking due to falls (to the side of the lesion), a nystagmus that may change direction and is not suppressed by visual fixation, the absence of hearing loss, and the presence of other neurological deficits are seen mostly in cerebellar strokes. Peripheral lesions, on the other hand, are associated with unidirectional nystagmus (with the fast component toward the normal ear) that does not reverse direction and is suppressed by visual fixation; less profound instability, associated hearing loss or tinnitus; and the absence of more neurological signs.[43] An MRI scan is the modality of choice for confirming or excluding posterior circulation stroke.

- In summary, the vast majority of patients presenting with vague dizziness or isolated vertigo symptoms will not have had a stroke and cerebellar ischaemic (established or transient) will be associated with ataxia and more pronounced symptoms.[44] In a recent *Lancet* review paper, it has been pointed out that cerebellar infarction can be difficult to diagnose because the clinical manifestations do not always raise concern. Vertebral dissection needs to always be considered and special note should be made of the timing patterns and triggers and not so much of the nature of dizziness or vertigo. If in doubt, do not hesitate to request an MRI, as misdiagnosis is common and mortality in this group is high.[45] Cerebellar infarction can simulate vestibular neuritis more commonly than previously thought, and vestibular neuritis is an important mimic that may lead to diagnostic pitfalls.[46]

- Brainstem ischaemia may result from occlusive disease affecting the vertebro-basilar circulation. This may be transient (TIA) or more permanent and involvement of the brainstem vestibular nuclei may lead to vertigo, but this is rarely the only symptom. Dysphagia, dysarthria, diplopia, gaze abnormalities, and intra-nuclear ophthalmoplegia are common with central lesions but are not seen in peripheral vestibulopathy. Imaging would reveal any established ischaemic foci, and a proportion of transiently ischaemic areas and angiography would identify occlusion.

- Lateral medullary infarction (also known as Wallenberg's syndrome) may result from occlusion or dissection of the ipsilateral vertebral artery. The latter supplies the lateral medulla via the branching posterior inferior cerebellar artery. Vertigo is seen, as well as ipsilateral Horner's, ipsilateral ataxia, abnormal eye movements, and a dissociated sensory loss (ipsilateral facial and contralateral truncal loss of pain and temperature). In other words, the clinical signs are profound, and imaging (MRI ± MRA) would uncover the underlying pathology.[47]

Sepsis

The systemic inflammatory response syndrome (SIRS) is central to sepsis and should satisfy at least two of the following features:

a Temperature > 38 °C or < 36 °C
b Tachycardia > 90 bpm
c Respiratory rate > 20 breaths per minute or $PaCO_2$ < 4.3 kPa
d WBC > 12 × 10^9/L or < 4 × 10^9/L, or > 10% immature (band) forms

Sepsis is SIRS in the presence of evidence of infection; severe sepsis implies organ hypoperfusion evident by, e.g., lactic acidosis, oliguria, or altered cerebral function; and septic shock entails hypotension (SBP < 90 mm Hg).

Sepsis is often included in literature reviews as a stroke mimic but should only rarely impose a diagnostic challenge. It is the altered cerebral function seen in severe sepsis that may manifest as reduced alertness, dysarthria, slurred speech, mutism, or acute confusional state. The latter is often the first sign of sepsis, especially in the elderly, but the true culprit should be easily uncovered by careful clinical observation, a screen for common causes of sepsis, and a thorough physical (including neurological) examination demonstrating no focal neurological deficits.

Infective endocarditis is a special case of sepsis and there are numerous historical reports of cerebral ischaemia, both established and transient, afflicting the anterior cerebral and vertebrobasilar vasculatures. In addition to embolic events, intraparenchymal and subarachnoid haemorrhage may also seen in infective endocarditis. Interestingly, TIA has even been reported to be the first and presenting complaint in infective endocarditis patients seeking medical attention, but this would be rare in our era.[48]

Toxic-metabolic encephalopathy

This is an aetiologically diverse clinical entity characterised by global cerebral dysfunction in the absence primary brain disease. More specific forms comprise:
- infectious
- hepatic
- uraemic
- hypoglycaemic
- Wernicke's
- hyponatraemic/hypernatraemic.

Decreased consciousness, dysphasia, tremor, fever, and abnormal reflexes are some common clinical features. Focal neurology, such as hemiparesis, may be seen with hypoglycaemia,[49] but generally focal deficits are absent. The clinical history, examination, and unrevealing neuro-imaging would be strong pointers to this diagnosis.

Space-occupying lesions

Space-occupying lesions, whether neoplastic or not, may present with a plethora of clinical manifestations, some of which may mimic stroke. These are presented in Table 8.5.

Tumours gradually increase in size but can cause neurological deficits of acute onset, especially where, for example, there has been bleeding into the tumour or a focal seizure. The deficit will vary depending on the anatomical location of the lesion and may not follow the pattern of vascular territory events. Brain imaging

TABLE 8.5 Clinical manifestations of brain masses

Generalised
 Headache
 Syncope
 Seizure
 Nausea and vomiting
 Cognitive impairment
Focal
 Dysphasia
 Hemiparesis
 Sensory loss
 Visual impairment

will assist with the diagnosis; sensitivity is required as the diagnosis will likely be unexpected.

A subdural haematoma may be regarded as a space-occupying lesion and may indeed be associated with focal neurological deficits but it very rarely presents a diagnostic challenge, especially if acute. The deficits result from the mechanical pressure that the haematinous mass exerts on adjacent brain structures. There are only rare reports of chronic subdural bleeds simulating TIA.[50] A history of brain trauma and confirmatory neuro-imaging would normally suffice for an accurate diagnosis.

Delirium
What is delirium?
The DSM-IV defines delirium as:
a   a disturbance of consciousness with reduced ability to focus, sustain, or shift attention;
b   a change in cognition or the development of a disturbance in perception that is not better accounted for by a pre-existing, established, or evolving dementia;
c   a disturbance that develops over a short period of time (usually hours to days) and tends to fluctuate during the course of the day;
d   Where there is evidence from the history, physical examination, or laboratory findings that the disturbance is caused by a medical condition, substance intoxication, or medication side effect.

Delirium and stroke
The problem arises from the fact that delirium is usually reasonably acute in onset and may appear to come on abruptly. This may be misinterpreted as sudden onset neurological deficit, which equals stroke or at least mandates stroke assessment.

Delirium may actually be the presenting feature of acute stroke and can complicate acute stroke in the early phase.[51] Recognising stroke as a concomitant or new feature in a stroke patient is important. Nevertheless, misdiagnosing one for the other should not occur too frequently as the clinical history on a par with clinical examination (which is revealing in stroke but unremarkable in pure delirium) would lead to accurate diagnosis.

Dementia

What is dementia?

The DSM-IV definition of dementia requires that the following criteria are met.

a   Evidence from the history and mental status examination showing major impairment in learning and memory as well as at least one of the following:
   –   impairment in the ability to handle complex tasks
   –   impairment in the ability to reason
   –   impaired spatial ability and impaired orientation
   –   impaired speech.
b   The cognitive symptoms significantly interfere with the individual's work performance, usual social activities, and relationships.
c   The decline from a previous level of functioning is significant.
d   The onset of the decline are of insidious onset and their course progressive, as evident from the clinical history or serial evaluations of mental status.
e   There is no concurrent delirium.
f   Psychiatric illness does not better explain the decline.
g   Systemic or brain disease is not thought to be better accountable for the decline.

Dementia and stroke

Dementia is a very distinct disorder and very occasionally might mimic stroke. The insidious onset and progressive course of dementia sets it apart. Misdiagnosis of dementia as stroke should consequently not happen if the above basic clinical definition is born in mind.

Vascular dementia, which is second after Alzheimer's in prevalence, is caused by large artery and lacunar infarction as well as chronic subcortical ischaemia. In other words, ischaemic stroke seems to the major causative factor of vascular dementia. Interestingly, the two entities do not seem to share the same cardiovascular risk factors.[52, 53] Their relation is certainly complex, and the precise pathobiology involved needs to be further researched and accurately elucidated.

Acute peripheral neuropathy

Any of the peripheral neuropathies, whether mononeuropathy, polyneuropathy, or mononeuropathy multiplex, may present acutely. Their causes vary from infectious and neoplastic to autoimmune and toxic and metabolic. Distinguishing peripheral from central lesions (stroke) should not present a diagnostic challenge and goes back to the basics of clinical history, neurological examination, and the presence or lack of relevant risk factors.

In the clinical history, the time course of the presenting complaint should be carefully explored. A sudden-onset deficit, not associated with pain, in an arteriopath of increased overall cardiovascular risk, makes stroke more likely. In such a case, the pattern of the deficit would follow an upper motor neuron pattern, with hyperreflexia, increased tone, a positive Babinski sign, weaker extensors in the upper limbs, and weak flexors in the lower limbs. Sensory loss would follow a wide central distribution and not a peripheral nerve one, such as that seen with peripheral nerve compression or entrapment (cf. carpal tunnel syndrome). Confirmatory diagnostic testing by means of appropriate imaging and the appropriate stroke work-up would provide further solid evidence of the clinical suspicion.

Spinal cord lesions

The majority of these in the acute setting are secondary to trauma and, despite the possible clinical resemblance to stroke, are readily recognised. The clinical pattern present would be immediately suggestive of the underlying lesion and imaging by computed tomography confirmatory.

Multiple sclerosis
Overview

Multiple sclerosis (MS) is a chronic inflammatory disease of the central nervous system of unknown cause with a prevalence of 1:1000 in the UK, a female preponderance (female to male ratio 2:1), and a tendency to present at 20–40 years. The clinical features are:
- *commonly visual*: decreased acuity, pain on eye movement, papillitis and optic atrophy on fundoscopy, relative afferent pupillary defect
- *sensory*: paraesthesiae, more loss of vibration and joint position sense than vibration and joint position sense
- *motor*: UMN signs, including hyperreflexia, spastic weakness, positive Babinski
- *cerebellar*: dysdiadochokinesis, dysmetria, past-pointing, cerebellar rebound, wide-based gait, scanning speech, uncoordinated heel-to-knee-to-heel test.

The diagnosis of MS relies on the identification of two or more CNS lesions with corresponding symptoms separated in time and space.

Stroke mimic?

There have been reports of MS presenting as stroke.[54, 55] Multiple sclerosis may present with acute deficits but the pattern of demyelination is very distinct, with visual and sensory symptoms predominating and a relapsing and remitting course. A high index of suspicion against stroke should alarm the physician when the history, the patient's age, the risk factor profile, and the examination are not typical of stroke.

Functional

The Hippocratic term *hysteria* (Greek for uterus) has been changed to conversion disorder and is recognised as a distinct psychiatric disorder. Blindness, deafness, hemiparesis, and hemiplegia are hysterical neurological manifestations that may mimic stroke. The lack of pattern in the symptoms present, the absence of risk factors for stroke and the presence of psychiatric illness in the past medical history may help uncover the neuropsychiatric origin of the presenting complaint easily.

IS IT REALLY A STROKE?

The main differences between stroke and the common and some of the less common mimics have been outlined above. In reality, distinguishing stroke from an imitator is an art and requires experience. Strategies for improving the diagnostic accuracy have been explored, and we shall herein discuss two landmark approaches.

The ROSIER scale

Nor and colleagues developed and validated the ROSIER scale, a clinical diagnostic scale aimed at assisting the accurate diagnosis of stroke in the A&E department. Diffusion-weighted MRI would be superior but this is not yet widely available in the acute setting, and stroke referrals rely on clinical acumen. The clinical scale developed uses clinical signs and has been shown to have a sensitivity of 93% at the cutoff point of +1.[56]

The brain attack study

Hand and colleagues identified 47 clinical factors that were found statistically significant in distinguishing a stroke from a mimic (*see* Table 8.6). Particularly strong

Assessment	Date	Time	
Symptom onset	Date	Time	
GCS	E =	M =	V =
BP =			
BM =			
(NB. If BM < 3–5 mmol/L, treat urgently and reassess once blood glucose is normal)			
Has there been loss of consciousness or syncope?		Y (–1)	N (0)
Has there been seizure activity?		Y (–1)	N (0)
Is there a NEW ACUTE onset (or on awakening from sleep)			
I. **Asymmetric facial weakness**		Y (+1)	N (0)
II. **Asymmetric arm weakness**		Y (+1)	N (0)
III. **Asymmetric leg weakness**		Y (+1)	N (0)
IV. **Speech disturbance**		Y (+1)	N (0)
V. **Visual field defect**		Y (+1)	N (0)
			*Total Score (-2 to +5)
Provisional diagnosis:	Stroke		Non-stroke (specify)
NB. Stroke is unlikely but not completely excluded if total scores are less than 0.			

FIGURE 8.1 The ROSIER scale *pro forma* (adapted from Nor, *et al.*)

TABLE 8.6 Factors in clinical assessment statistically significant in predicting stroke

VARIABLE
Past medical history
  Cognitive impairment
  Ischaemic heart disease
  Peripheral vascular disease
Presenting complaint
  Exact time of onset
  Recall onset
  Well last week
  Can walk now
  Lost consciousness
  Headache
  Seizure at onset
  Definite focal symptoms
  Visual loss
  Loss of speech/language
  Sensory loss—face
  Weakness—arm
  Sensory loss—arm
  Weakness—hand
  Sensory loss—hand
  Weakness—leg
  Sensory loss—leg
  No lateralising symptoms
General examination
  SBP > 150 mm Hg
  DBP > 90 mm Hg
  Heart murmur
  Signs in other systems
  Confusion
Neurological examination
  Abnormal verbal output
  Slurred speech
  Hemianopia
  Visual inattention
  Eye deviation
  Facial asymmetry
  Arm weakness
  Hand weakness
  Leg weakness
  Sensory loss
  Visuospatial dysfunction
  Upper limb ataxia
  Extensor plantar
  No neurological signs

(Continued)

TABLE 8.6 Factors in clinical assessment statistically significant in predicting stroke (*Continued*)

Diagnostic Formulation
No lateralising signs
Signs inconsistent with symptoms
Signs not equal vascular territory
OCSP – TACS
OCSP – LACS
OCSP – Unsure

(Adapted from Hand, et al.)

predictors were the presence of focal symptoms, the patient's well status in the week preceding the 'brain attack', and an easily determined exact time of onset.[57]

Vertigo and limb ataxia were more likely to predict a mimic (non-stroke vestibulopathy). Loss of consciousness, seizure at onset, the absence of lateralising symptoms, the presence of confusion, discrepancy between signs and symptoms, and the presence of other physical signs but no neurological signs were all found to be pointers to a mimic than an actual stroke.[57]

The National Institute of Health Stroke Scale was useful in distinguishing mimic from stroke, but 19% of cases with a score of more than 10 were found to be attributable to a mimic.[57]

The identified clinical factors can assist in the more accurate diagnosis and complements laboratory testing and imaging in the emergency department[57] but, of course, clinical experience is indispensable to the process.

REFERENCES

1. Hand PJ, Kwan J, Lindley RI, *et al*. Distinguishing between stroke and mimic at the bedside: the brain attack study. *Stroke*. 2006; **37**(3): 769–75.
2. Libman RB, Wirkowski E, Alvir J, *et al*. Conditions that mimic stroke in the emergency department. Implications for acute stroke trials. *Arch Neurol*. 1995; **52**(11): 1119–22.
3. Azlisham MN, Davis J, Sen B, *et al*. The Recognition of Stroke in the Emergency Room (ROSIER) scale: development and validation of a stroke recognition instrument. *Lancet Neurol*. 2005; **4**: 727–34.
4. Hatzitolios A, Savopoulos C, Ntaios G, *et al*. Stroke and conditions that mimic it: a protocol secures a safe early recognition. *Hippokratia*. 2008; **12**(2): 98–102.
5. Flossmann E, Redgrave JN, Briley D, *et al*. Reliability of clinical diagnosis of the symptomatic vascular territory in patients with recent transient ischemic attack or minor stroke. *Stroke*. 2008; **39**(9): 2457–60.
6. Scher AI, Launer LJ. Migraine: Migraine with aura increases the risk of stroke. *Nat Rev Neurol*. 2010; **6**(3): 128–9.
7. Cutler FM, Moskowitz MA. Headaches and other head pain. In: Goldman L, Ausiello D, editors. *Cecil Textbook of Medicine*. 22nd ed. Saunders; 2004.

8. Raskin NH. Headache. In: Kasper DL, Braunwald E, Fauci A, *et al.*, editors. *Harrison's Principles of Internal Medicine*. 16th ed. McGraw-Hill; 2005.

9. Mishra NK, Rossetti AO, Ménétrey A, *et al.* Recurrent Wernicke's aphasia: migraine and not stroke! *Headache.* 2009; **49**(5): 765–8.

10. Fisher CM. Late-life migraine accompaniments as a cause of unexplained transient ischemic attacks. *Can J Neurol Sci.* 1980; **7**: 9.

11. Lempert T, Neuhauser H. Vertigo as a symptom of migraine. *Med Klin* (Munich). 2001; **96**(8): 475–9.

12. Grosberg B, Solomon S, Friedman D, *et al.* Retinal migraine reappraised. *Cephalalgia.* 2006; **26**: 1275.

13. Ducros A. Familial and sporadic hemiplegic migraine. *Rev Neurol* (Paris). 2008; **164**(3): 216–24.

14. Headache Classification Subcommittee of the International Headache Society. The international classification of headache disorders. 2nd ed. *Cephalalgia.* 2004; **24** Suppl 1: 9.

15. Lipton RB, Bigal ME, Steiner TJ, *et al.* Classification of primary headaches. *Neurology.* 2004; **63**: 427.

16. Bickerstaff ER. The basilar artery and the migraine-epilepsy syndrome. *Proc R Soc Med.* 1962; **55**: 167–9.

17. Perkin GD. Epilepsy in later childhood and adults. In: Warrel DA, Cox TM, Firth JD, *et al.*, editors. *Oxford Textbook of Medicine.* 4th ed. Oxford University Press; 2006.

18. Fuller G, Manford M. Epilepsy I: diagnosis. In: *Neurology: an illustrated colour text.* 2nd ed. Churchill Livingstone (Elsevier); 2006.

19. Todd RB. *Clinical lectures on paralysis, certain diseases of the brain, and other affections of the nervous system.* John Churchill; 1854: 284–307.

20. Rolak LA, Rutecki P, Ashizawa T, *et al.* Clinical features of Todd's post-epileptic paralysis. *J Neurol Neurosurg Psych.* 1992; **55**: 63–4.

21. Rupprecht S, Schwab M, Fitzek C, *et al.* Hemispheric hypoperfusion in postictal paresis mimics early brain ischaemia. *Epilepsy Res.* 2010; **89**(2–3): 355–9.

22. Glick TH. The sleep-deprived electroencephalogram: evidence of practice. *Arch Neurol.* 2002; **59**: 1235.

23. King MA, Newton MR, Jackson GD, *et al.* Epileptology of the first seizure presentation: a clinical, electroencephalographic, and magnetic resonance imaging study of 300 consecutive patients. *Lancet.* 1998; **352**: 1007.

24. Marsan CA, Zivin LS. Factors related to the occurrence of typical paroxysmal abnormalities in the EEG records of epileptic patients. *Epilepsia.* 1970; **11**: 361.

25. van Donselaar CA, Schimscheimer RJ, Geerts AT, *et al.* Value of the electroencephalogram in adult patients with untreated idiopathic first seizure. *Arch Neurol.* 1992; **49**: 231.

26. Zivin L, Marsan CA. Incidence and prognostic significance of 'epileptiform' activity in the EEG of non-epileptic subjects. *Brain.* 1968; **91**: 751.

27. Bridgers SL. Epileptiform abnormalities discovered on electroencephalographic screening of psychiatric inpatients. *Arch Neurol.* 1987; **44**: 312.

28. Bladin CF, Alexandrov AV, Bellavance A, *et al.* Seizures after stroke: a prospective multicenter study. *Arch Neurol.* 2000; **57**(11): 1617–22.

29. Richardson EP, Dodge PR. Epilepsy in cerebrovascular disease. *Epilepsia.* 1954; **3**: 49–65.

30. Aring CD, Merritt HH. Differential dignosis between cerebral haemorrhage and cerebral thrombosis; clinical and pathological study of 245 cases. *Arch Int Med.* 1935; **56**: 435–56.

31. Louis S, McDowell F. Epileptic seizures in non-embolic cerebral infarction. *Arch Neurol.* 1967; **17**: 414–18.

32. Brognole M, Alboni P, Benditt D. Guidelines on management, and treatment of syncope. *Eur Heart J.* 2001; **22**: 1256–306.

33. Kapoor WN. Syncope. *N Engl J Med.* 2000; **343**: 1856–62.

34. Davidson E, Rotenbeg Z, Fuchs J, *et al.* Transient ischaemic attack-related syncope. *Clin Cardiol.* 1991; **14**: 141–4.

35. Hand RJ, Kwan J, Lindley RI. Distinguishing between stroke and a mimic at the bedside: the brain attack study. *Stroke.* 2006; **37**: 769–75.

36. Bartsch T, Deuschl G. Transient global amnesia: functional anatomy and clinical implications. *Lancet Neurol.* 2010; **9**: 205–14.

37. Hodges JR, Warlow CP. Syndromes of transient amnesia: towards a classification. A study of 153 cases. *J Neurol Neurosurg Psychiatry.* 1990; **53**: 834–43.

38. Crossman AR, Neary D. Cranial nerves and cranial nerve nuclei. *Neuroanatomy: an illustrated colour text.* 2nd ed. Churchill Livingstone; 2004.

39. Froehling DA, Silverstein MD, Mohr DN, *et al.* Benign positional vertigo: incidence and prognosis in a population-based study in Olmsted County, Minnesota. *Mayo Clin Proc.* 1991; **66**: 596.

40. Zingler VC, Weintz E, Jahn K, *et al.* Follow-up of vestibular function in bilateral vestibulopathy. *J Neurol Neurosurg Psychiatry.* 2008; **79**: 284.

41. Frohman EM, Zhang H, Dewey RB, *et al.* Vertigo in MS: utility of positional and particle repositioning maneuvers. *Neurology.* 2000; **55**: 1566.

42. Baloh RW, Yue Q, Furman JM, *et al.* Familial episodic ataxia: Clinical heterogeneity in four families linked to chromosome 19p. *Ann Neurol.* 1997; **41**: 8.

43. Hotson JR, Baloh RW. Acute vestibular syndrome. *N Engl J Med.* 1998; **339**: 680.

44. Kerber KA, Brown DL, Lisabeth LD, *et al.* Stroke among patients with dizziness, vertigo, and imbalance in the emergency department: a population-based study. *Stroke.* 2006; **37**(10): 2484–7.

45. Edlow JA, Newman-Toker DE, Savitz SI. Diagnosis and initial management of cerebellar infarction. *Lancet Neurol.* 2008; **7**(10): 951–6.

46. Lee H, Sohn SI, Cho YW, *et al.* Cerebellar infarction presenting with isolated vertigo: frequency and vascular topographical patterns. *Neurology.* 2006; **67**: 1178–83.

47. Fisher CM, Karnes WE, Kubik CS. Lateral medullary infarction: the pattern of vascular occlusion. *J Neuropathol Exp Neurol.* 1961; **20**: 323.

48. Jones HR, Siekert RG. Neurological manifestations of infective endocarditis; review of clinical and therapeutic challenges. *Brain.* 1989; **112**: 1295–315.

49. Malouf R, Brust JC. Hypoglycaemia: causes, neurological manifestations and outcome. *Ann Neurol.* 1985; **17**(5): 421–30.

50. Ribó M, Montaner J, Molina C, *et al.* Chronic subdural hematoma simulating a TIA. *Neurologia.* 2002; **17**(6): 342–4.

51. Oldenbeuving AW, de Kort PL, Jansen BP, *et al.* Delirium in acute stroke: a review. *Int J Stroke.* 2007; **2**(4): 270–5.

52. Potluri R, Natalwala A, Uppal H, *et al.* Different risk factors in vascular dementia and ischaemic stroke. *Neuroepidemiology.* 2009; **32**(1): 80.

53. Iemolo F, Duro G, Rizzo C, *et al*. Patho-physiology of vascular dementia. *Immun Ageing*. 2009; **6**: 13.
54. Norris JW, Hachinski JC. Misdiagnosis of stroke. *Lancet*. 1982; **319**(8267): 328–31.
55. Qui W, Wu J-S, Carroll WM, *et al*. Wallenberg syndrome caused by multiple sclerosis mimicking stroke. *J Clin Neurosc*. 2009; **16**(12): 1700–02.
56. Nor AM, Davis J, Sen B, *et al*. The Recognition of Stroke in the Emergency Room (ROSIER) scale: development and validation of a stroke recognition instrument. *Lancet Neurol*, 2005; **4**: 727–34.
57. Hand PJ, Kwan J, Lindley RI, *et al*. Distinguishing between stroke and mimic at the bedside. *Stroke*. 2006; **37**: 769–75.

CHAPTER 9

Stroke in young people

INTRODUCTION

While generally viewed as a disease of the elderly, stroke may also affect children and young adults. Presentation with stroke is rare in these groups, and the underlying causes differ from those seen in more elderly patients. This chapter will review the ways in which cerebrovascular disease may affect young people and discuss how the investigation and management of stroke differs in the young compared to the elderly.

EPIDEMIOLOGY

Stroke in young adults is rare (the annual incidence in adults under 45 years is estimated to lie between 4 and 11 cases per 100 000) and rarer still in children, where the annual incidence rate is between 1 and 8 cases per 100 000 per year. Conventional risk factors for stroke such as cigarette smoking, hypertension, and dyslipidaemia are less common in children and young adults, and factors such as congenital heart disease, blood disorders such as sickle-cell disease and thrombophilias, abuse of illicit substances, and genetic and metabolic disorders are more frequently implicated in the pathogenesis of stroke.

Important risk factors for stroke in children
Sickle-cell disease

Sickle-cell disease confers a high risk of stroke throughout the patient's lifetime and is a particularly important cause of stroke during childhood. Haemoglobin S (Hb S) is an abnormal form of haemoglobin caused by a single gene mutation. The mutation causes a single amino acid substitution on the globin beta chain. This substitution causes the haemoglobin within red blood corpuscles to polymerise when exposed to low oxygen tension. The polymerisation of haemoglobin causes the red corpuscles to become stiffer and less pliable, reducing their ability to pass through capillary beds.

The most clamant clinical manifestation of sickle-cell disease is a propensity to acute 'crises' characterised by diffuse pain, haemolysis, and worsening of anaemia. Other problems faced by sufferers include greater susceptibility to infection due to splenic dysfunction and a higher risk of vascular events.

The cerebrovascular sequelae of sickle-cell disease may arise through a number of mechanisms. Patients frequently have evidence of small vessel ischaemia on brain imaging, which may be asymptomatic and presumably caused by tissue hypoperfusion due to impacted red cells in the capillary beds. In addition, fibrous proliferation of the intimal layers of larger intra- and extracranial vessels may occur, causing stenosis or occlusion. This may lead to territorial infarction of the brain, and in some cases, cerebral haemorrhage may occur from the fragile network of collateral vessels that can form in response to occlusion of the larger intracranial vessels (see moyamoya disease).

There is no specific therapy for sickle-cell-related stroke: management of crises includes oxygenation and exchange transfusion. In the longer term, vascular complications including stroke may be minimised by prophylactic exchange transfusion and hydroxycarbamide therapy, which reduces the proportion of circulating abnormal haemoglobin.

Heart disease

Structural cardiac abnormalities, particularly those involving abnormal communication between cardiac chambers with the risk of paradoxical embolism, confer elevated risk of stroke. Children may develop stroke either as a direct consequence of the structural abnormality or as a complication of surgical intervention to treat it.

Abnormalities of the cerebral vasculature

Abnormalities of the cerebral vessels, either inherited or acquired, may predispose to stroke in childhood. Some, such as moyamoya, arterial dissection, and vasculitis, share a common pathogenesis with adults and are discussed later. Others, such as focal cerebral arteriopathy of childhood and postvaricella encephalopathy, are more specifically associated with childhood stroke.

Focal cerebral arteriopathy of childhood (FCA)

FCA is a term used to describe an idiopathic stenotic lesion in a cerebral artery causing stroke in a child. Although its aetiology is obscure and probably multifactorial, an association with recent upper respiratory tract infection has been described. Serial imaging studies have shown partial or complete resolution in a proportion of affected individuals, implying a reversible, but as-yet-unelucidated mechanism.

Postvaricella encephalopathy

This condition is felt to be distinct from FCA, with a better-defined phenotype involving focal stenosis of the proximal middle cerebral artery with distal infaction, occurring in the context of recent varicella infection.

Mitochondrial encephalopathy with lactic acidosis and stroke-like episodes (MELAS)

MELAS is a rare disorder of mitochondrial DNA that presents with recurrent episodes of stroke-like focal neurological disturbance in childhood or adolescence.[1] Over time, the cumulative effect of these recurrences may lead to progressive disability and cognitive impairment, which may be compounded by other clinical features characteristic of mitochondrial disorders, such as proximal muscle weakness and ataxia. Migraine, seizures, and sensorineural deafness may also occur.

The diagnosis of MELAS can be made thorough examination of mitochondrial DNA, although not all mutations are readily identifiable by current techniques. Supporting evidence for the diagnosis may be obtained from brain imaging (typically changes consistent with occipital infarction on MR imaging, with marked radiological improvement over subsequent weeks) and on MR spectroscopy, which may show elevation of brain lactate concentration. CSF analysis shows a similar rise in lactate, and muscle biopsy may show characteristic 'ragged red fibres'. Treatment is supportive and includes provision of non-pharmacological measures such as physiotherapy and hearing aids, together with anticonvulsant treatment where appropriate.

Presentation of stroke in children

Presentation of stroke in children may differ from presentation in adults. While both groups frequently present with the abrupt onset of focal neurological symptoms and signs, younger children and infants may develop a less-specific syndrome involving altered mental state of seizure activity. The less-specific nature of the presentation may obscure, complicate, and delay the diagnosis.

Risk factors for stroke in young adults
Arterial dissection

Dissection of the carotid and vertebral arteries is a common cause of stroke in young people, accounting for about 10% of all strokes in those under 45 years of age. Dissection of an artery occurs following a tear in the initmal layer of the vessel, allowing blood to penetrate the arterial wall. The blood may track between tissue planes withn the artery, creating a 'false' lumen, narrowing the true lumen and causing a characteristic angiographic appearance. This process typically causes craniofacial pain, and distortion of the affected vessel may cause compression of adjacent structures causing local peripheral neurological symptoms and signs; however, approximately one-third of all dissections present with cerebrovascular syndromes.

Most arterial dissections occur in the extracranial portion of the carotid and vertebral arteries. In about half of all cases, a history of trauma is apparent, which may
be relatively minor. Cases of arterial dissection have, for example, been reported
following neck extension at the hairdresser.

Those with conditions characterised by connective tissue abnormalities such as
Ehlers-Danlos syndrome are at elevated risk of dissection and recurrence, as are
patients with disordered arterial anatomy such as fibromuscular dysplasia. It is
possible that more minor disorders of collagen and connective tissue could confer
elevated risk of dissection, but these are not routinely sought.

Due to the frequency with which dissection causes stroke in the young, it should
be considered in the differential diagnosis of any young patient, particularly those
with characteristic pain or a history of neck trauma. Characteristic features should
be sought from the history and examination of all such patients.

The presence of craniofacial or cervical pain is highly suggestive of dissection;
this may occur days or even weeks before the onset of any neurological deficit and
is typically ipsilateral to the dissection. Features that should raise suspicion of a
carotid artery dissection include ipsilateral Horner's syndrome and less commonly
lower cranial nerve palsies (IX, X, and XII) caused by local compression of these
nerves as they run adjacent to the damaged artery. Vertebral arterial dissection tends
not to cause cranial neuropathy but is typically associated with posterior neck and
occipital pain.

In all cases where dissection is suspected, imaging of the neck vessels should
be undertaken without delay. Unfortunately, carotid ultrasound has only limited
sensitivity to detect arterial dissection, although in some cases, a dissection flap of
damaged intima may be visualised. Cross-sectional techniques are superior to ultrasound in this regard, and magnetic resonance angiography is the preferred modality. Magnetic resonance angiography reveals the characteristic tapered or occluded
appearance of a dissected artery, and axial fat-suppressed sequences, a bright area of
high signal, can be detected within the wall of the vessel, indicating the presence of
blood in the false lumen.

There is a paucity of evidence to guide then management of patients with stroke
secondary to arterial dissection: most guidelines recommend anticoagulation for
between three and six months until recanalisation occurs. There is no evidence
that antiplatelet treatment alone is inferior to this approach, and comparative trials to inform future management are underway. The prognosis is generally good,
with a low lifetime risk of recurrent dissection in those without an underlying
predisposition.

Drug abuse

Illicit drug use should be considered in all young patients with stroke, and urine
screening for drugs of abuse undertaken in all cases where it is suspected as a potential aetiological factor. Sympathomimetic drugs such as cocaine and amphetamines[2]

cause marked and aprupt increases in blood pressure and may precipitate cerebral vasospasm or, through a mechanism that has yet to be elucidated, cerebral vasculitis. Both drugs have been associated with cerebral infaction and cerebral haemorrhage following recreational use. Intravenous abuse of any drug poses a risk of stroke through infective endocarditis due to non-sterile technique, paradoxical embolism of particulate matter or cerebral hypoperfusion following drug-induced hypotension.

Cerebral vasculitis

Inflammation of the cerebral vasculature may occur as part of a broad spectrum of focal and systemic disorders, involving any size of intracranial vessel and causing a wide variety of clinical presentations, including stroke. This section will discuss the vasculitides that may present to a stroke unit, stratified by the size of the vessel involved.

Large vessel vasculitis

Temporal arteritis

In contrast to many other vasculitic disorders, temporal arteritis is primarily a condition of the elderly and is very rare in those under 60 years of age. Although almost any vessel can be affected, there is a predeliction for the ophthalmic artery and the branches of the external carotid artery. Accordingly, patients with temporal arteritis may present to stroke services with monocular blindness. There should be a low index of suspicion for temporal arteritis in all elderly patients with transient monocular blindness as prompt identification and treatment may prevent progression to permanent visual loss. Associated features may include tenderness over the temporal arteries and evidence of ischaemia in the territory supplied by the external carotid artery, with claudication of the jaw being the best-recognised clinical manifestation. Definitive diagnosis is by temporal artery biopsy, which reveals patchy granulomatous inflammation. ESR is usually markedly elevated, and liver function tests may be mildly deranged. Features of the related condition giant cell arteritis (fatigue, proximal muscle weakness, and stiffness) may also be present. As the condition may progress rapidly with the prospect of permanent visual loss, treatment with high dose corticosteroids is recommended before a definitive pathological diagnosis is obtained.

Takayasu's arteritis

This is a rare large vessel vasculitis that occurs most commonly in young women, particularly those of Asian descent. It affects the great vessels as they arise from the aortic arch, causing inflammation, stenosis, and eventually occlusion. Presentation is usually with symptoms of focal ischaemia or brain or upper limbs, although the coronary, renal, and occasionally lower limb arteries can be affected. Characteristic angiographic appearances are sufficient to make the diagnosis in patients with an appropriate clinical presentation, and treatment is with corticosteroids.

Intermediate vessel vasculitis

Isolated vasculitis of the central nervous system

This is an unusual granulomatous vasculitis confined, by definition, to the CNS, which predominantly affects medium-sized and small cerebral vessels. There are few if any peripheral markers of the condition; however, ESR may occasionally be elevated. It may present as an encephalopathy or as recurrent stroke, particularly affecting white matter. Normal cerebral angiography does not exclude the condition as the inflammatory change may be confined to very small vessels that are not well-visualised by current techniques. Lymphocytic pleocytosis may occur and is supportive of the diagnosis, but this is not a universal finding. Isolated vasculitis of the central nervous system is a rare condition whose diagnosis of is fraught with difficulty. Evidence to guide management is lacking, but most authorities advocate immunosuppressive therapy.

Polyarteritis nodosa (PAN)

PAN is a systemic necrotising vasculitis that tends to affect medium-sized arteries, including the cerebral arteries. Involvement of these arteries causes ischaemic stroke or TIA, which may be the presenting feature or which may occur in the context of multi-organ involvement. Associated features include constitutional symptoms such as generalised myalgia and weight loss, mononeuropathies are common, and there may be renal and/or cardiac involvement. The diagnosis is based upon clinical features supported by laboratory evience of antineutrophil cytoplasmic antibodies (ANCA) and an eosinophilia in peripheral blood. The symptoms usually respond swiftly to aggressive immunosuppressant therapy.

Wegener's granulomatosis

This is a condition related to PAN, which also causes systemic inflammation of small- and medium-sized vessels. Involvement of the respiratory tract and kidney are common, with granulomatous inflammation causing nasal inflammation and ulceration, abnormalities on chest radiograph, and evidence of glomerulonephritis. Other vascular beds, including the cerebral circulation, may be involved. As with PAN, immunosuppressive therapy is the mainstay of treatment.

Systemic lupus erythematosus (SLE)

SLE may present with stroke through a variety of mechanisms, including the induction of a prothrombotic state, an association with cardiac valvular inflammation (Liebman-Sachs endocarditis), and an association with cerebral vasculitis. The cerebral vasculitis of SLE may cause stroke; however, more common clinical manifestations include vasculitis-related encephalopathy, neuropsychiatric syndromes, and seizure.

Cerebral autosomal dominant arteropathy with subcortical infarcts and leucoencephalopathy (CADASIL)

CADASIL is a systemic disease of the vasculature whose clinical effects are confined to the brain.[3] Its name encapsulates the key clinical and radiological features of the condition. It is associated with mutations in the notch 3 gene that codes for a transmembrane protein involved in intercellular signalling. The phenotype is variable; however, in typical cases, affected patients remain symptom-free until the third decade of life, when they develop migrainous symptoms, usually with aura. Subcortical stroke occurs in the fourth and fifth decades, with subsequent dementia and occasionally an associated depressive illness and/or seizure disorder. The distinctive clinical picture should raise suspicion of CADASIL, and a careful family history is an essential component of the evaluation. Relatives of an affected patient may have been misdiagnosed with other causes of progressive neurological symptoms, such as multiple sclerosis or Alzheimer's disease, and this should be borne in mind. CADASIL is associated with distinctive magnetic resonance appearances, characteristically widespread white matter disease with particular involvement of the temporal poles. Genetic testing is now available, and many of the mutations in the notch 3 gene have been identified. Given the progressive nature of the condition and the absence of specific therapeutic options, appropriate counselling should always be undertaken before the genetic tests are performed.

Management is essentially supportive, with modification of vascular risk factors, antiplatelet therapy following stroke, and both anticonvulsant and antidepressant therapy as necessary.

Fabry's disease

Fabry's disease is a rare, x-linked recessive disorder charcterised by relative deficiency of the enzyme alpha-galactosidase A. Lack of this enzyme causes the accumulation of glycosphingolipids in a wide variety of tissues, including peripheral nerves, blood vessels, and cardiac muscle. The clinical features of Fabry's disease are therefore rather diverse, and it may present a diagnostic challenge to a broad spectrum of clinicians.

Within the cerebral vasculature, Fabry's disease may cause small vessel dysfunction, white matter ischaemia, and lacunar cerebral infarction.[4] Glycospingolipid accumulation within the walls of larger arteries (particularly the vertebrobasilar vessels) may also cause territorial infarction. Diagnosis of Fabry's disease is predicated upon genetic testing or measurement of alpha-galactosidase enzyme activity and is not routinely performed. Prevalence of Fabry's disease among young patients with cryptogenic stroke is uncertain, but some early reports suggest approximately 1 in 20 such patients may be affected.

Patients with Fabry's disease may complain of neurpathic pain related to involvement of peripheral sensory nerves, and cardiac manifestations including hypertrophy of cardiac muscle may be apparent. Enzyme replacement therapy is now available for patients with Fabry's disease, but the effect of this treatment on risk of stroke is unknown.

Thrombophilia

The thrombophilias are a hererogeneous group of disorders, both inherited and acquired, which predispose to the development of thrombosis. The relationship between thrombophilia and stroke is contentious and requires further study.

The most common inherited thrombophilia is the Factor V Leiden mutation, present in approximately 5% of the adult population. This polymorphism leads to the creation of a form of Factor V that is resistant to cleavage by the activated form of the endogenous anticoagulant protein C. Resistance to activated protein C is associated with venous thrombosis; however, the relationship with arterial thrombosis and ischaemic stroke is less clear.

Overt deficiency of endogenous anticoagulant proteins such as protein C or protein S also predisoposes to the development of thrombosis. These deficiencies may be inherited or acquired, and a weak association with young stroke has been reported. Levels of proteins C and S may fluctuate and are known to fall in the context of acute illness such as stroke. For this reason, a convalescent sample is usually recommended before the diagnosis can be confirmed.

If a causal relationship is suspected between stroke and deficiency of proteins C or S, or resistance to activated protein C, lifelong anticoagulation is usually initiated.

Anticardiolipin antibodies are antibodies that bind to phospholipids. They may occur in patients with SLE, malignancy or chronic infection, and as part of the anticardiolipin antibody syndrome, which comprises a tendency to both arterial and venous thrombosis, recurrent miscarriage, thrombocytopenia, cardiac valve vegetations, and the characteristic skin rash ('livedo reticularis'). Once identified, patients with the anticardiolipin antibody syndrome are anticoagulated for life.

Specific considerations in young women
Oral contraceptive pill (OCP) and stroke

Oral contraceptive preparations may be associated with a minor excess risk of stroke. This modest risk, not reproduced in all epidemiological studies, would appear to be confined to ischemic stroke and the use of the combined oral contraceptive pill. The absolute risk in healthy young (< 35 years) women without significant vascular risk factors is very low[5] and is not usually an influential factor when contraceptive use is planned. Use of OCP by older women with vascular risk factors would appear to carry greater risk and is generally not recommended. OCP use in these women should be considered on a case-by-case basis.

Stroke in pregnancy

Pregnant women and those in the puerperium are at elevated risk of stroke.[6] The major contributors to this elevated risk are the linked conditions of preeclampsia,

eclampsia, and HELLP (hemolysis, elevated liver enzymes, and low platelets) that constitute the more frequently encountered causes of cerebral haemorrhage and infarction. Although they are strongly associated with stroke, the neurovascular manifestations of these conditions more frequently present with an encephalo-pathic syndrome with headache, visual disturbance, obtundation, and seizures.

The risk of stroke in pregnancy is further augmented by postpartum angiopathy, which is characterised by severe headache and focal neurological signs arising as a consequence of intense cerebral vasospasm. Some authorities consider postpartum angiopathy to be a variant of eclampsia.

Management of these conditions is directed towards prevention of seizures, low-ering of blood pressure to reduce risk of cerebral haemorrhage, to promptly deliver the infant, and to stabilise the mother.

Pregnancy is an hypercoagulable state, with progressive resistance to activated protein C developing in the second half of gestation, together with a reduction in activity of fibrinolysis inhibitors and an increased concentration of circulat-ing clotting factors. These factors generally predispose to venous thrombosis and may interact with a pre-existing thrombophilic tendency. Most authorities recom-mend exclusion of an underlying acquired or inherited thrombophilia in pregnant patients with ischaemic stroke.

Stroke in pregnancy is usually investigated and treated in a similar fashion to non-pregnant individuals. Brain imaging with magnetic resonance is preferred where feasible due to its greater sensitivity and lack of exposure to ionising radia-tion. Acute management strategies are more limited as recent delivery is regarded as an absolute contraindication to thrombolytic therapy. There is a paucity of evidence to inform the use of thrombolytic therapy during pregnancy; however, guidelines recommend the avoidance of such intervention given the potential risk of haem-orrhage. Secondary preventative strategies should be targeted at the likely mecha-nism and counselling on risk of stroke during future pregnancy should be provided. This risk is determined by the mechanistic basis of the stroke but is generally low, with most studies suggesting a recurrence rate approximating to 1%, suggesting that stroke during pregnancy should not be regarded as a contraindication to future pregnancies.

REFERENCES

1. Pavlakis SG, Phillips PC, DiMauro S, *et al*. Mitochondrial myopathy, encephalop-athy, lactic acidosis and strokelike episodes: a distinctive clinical syndrome. *Ann Neurol*. 1984; **16**: 481–8.
2. Heye N, Hankey GJ. Amphetamine-associated stroke. *Cerebrovasc Dis*. 1996; **6**: 149–55.
3. Kalimo H, Ruchoux MM, Viitanen M, *et al*. CADASIL: a common form of heredi-tary arteriopathy causing brain infarcts and dementia. *Brain Pathol*. 2002; **12**: 371–84.

4. Moore DF, Kaneski CR, Askari H, *et al.* The cerebral vasculopathy of Fabry disease. *J Neurol Sci.* 2007; **257**: 258.
5. Bousser MG, Kittner SJ. Oral contraceptives and stroke. *Cephalalgia.* 2000; **20**: 183–9.
6. Davie CA, O'Brien P. Stroke and pregnancy. *J Neurol Neurosurg Psychiatry.* 2008; **79**: 240–5.

FURTHER READING

• Caplan LR, Bogousslavsky J, editors. *Uncommon Causes of Stroke.* Cambridge University Press; 2008.

CHAPTER 10

An aid to neuroimaging

INTRODUCTION

Neuroimaging serves several purposes in acute stroke. Its prime purpose is to enable rapid differentiation of ischaemic from haemorrhagic stroke and to exclude important mimics such as tumour and subdural haematoma. Imaging also serves to identify lesion location and helps establish aetiology of stroke. This chapter will describe the basic principles of CT, MRI, and ultrasound imaging and how these modalities are used and interpreted in the evaluation of acute stroke.

BASIC PRINCIPLES OF COMPUTED TOMOGRAPHY SCANNING

Computed tomography (CT) scanning is an x-ray based technique. CT scanners incorporate an x-ray source that rotates around the patient, directing the x-rays toward the part of the body being scanned. The degree of absorption of x-rays increases with increasing density of body tissues. Non-absorbed x-rays pass through the body and fall upon a radiation detector, and the number hitting the detector is recorded and provides an index of body tissue density. A reconstruction phase allows this information to be expressed as a picture where tissues of the highest density appear bright (white) and those of lowest density appear dark (black).

The relative densities of tissues are expressed as Hounsfield units (HU). The HU scale runs from −1000 (air: lowest density, lowest absorption, and appears black) to >1000 (dense bone: highest density, highest absorption, and appears bright white), although most body tissues lie in the range of −100 to 100 and most cranial CT scanners specifically study tissues within this more restricted range. Just as the differences between density of body tissues allows them to be distinguished from each other, the changes in tissue composition that follow cerebral infarction and haemorrhage allow these lesions to be detected and to some extent aged. For example, an acute influx of water to neuronal cells and cytotoxic oedema follows onset of cerebral ischaemia. Vasogenic oedema may follow and ultimately tissue infarction will occur, and after several months, the infarcted area is entirely transformed into a fluid-filled space. Following intracerebral haemorrhage, dense congealed blood appears within the brain parenchyma, and again, over a prolonged period, this area is also transformed into a fluid-filled space.

CT TECHNIQUES USED IN ACUTE STROKE

A non-contrast enhanced CT (NCCT) brain scan will provide enough diagnostic information in many patients. This usually contains images of 10 or 11 transverse slices of brain tissue and can be acquired rapidly. On a NCCT scan of the brain, the highly dense and thus bright white skull bones can easily be seen enclosing the brain. Other areas of calcification, such as that within the ventricles, are commonly seen and are normal. The junction of the gray and white matter in the brain can be seen, as white matter is slightly less dense and therefore darker in appearance than gray matter. Similarly, the subcortical nuclei are visible, as they are slightly lighter in appearance than the surrounding gray matter and adjacent ventricles. The ventricles are the darkest structures on the scan as they are fluid-filled. An example from a normal slice of brain tissue on NCCT is shown in Figure 10.1.

Infarcted brain tissue, because of increased water content, appears as an area of reduced density and is darker or hypoattenuated relative to surrounding tissue. Oedema is limited in the early hours after onset of ischaemic stroke and thus acute infarction is often not visible on NCCT for several hours. Early signs of these changes include sulcal asymmetry and loss of gray-white matter differentiation, including in the basal ganglia where the subcortical nuclei may be obscured and

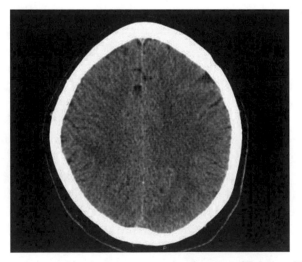

FIGURE 10.1 Slice of normal brain tissue on a non-contrast CT scan of brain. The highly dense bone is readily seen, as is the grey-white matter junction

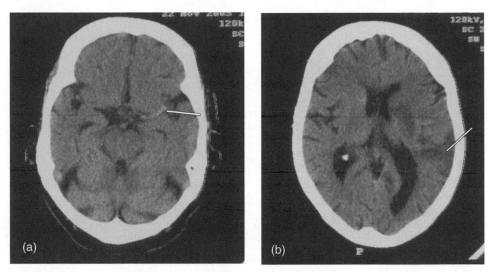

FIGURE 10.2 A dense left middle cerebral artery sign (arrow) and an area of cerebral infarction at 24 hours after thrombolytic therapy (non-contrast brain CT)

in the insular ribbon (the insular sign). Further, in acute middle cerebral artery thrombosis, a hyperdense middle cerebral artery may be visible immediately after onset (*see* Figure 10.2). After 24 to 48 hours, the area of hypoattenuation becomes obvious (*see* Figure 10.2) and ultimately, as the infarcted area becomes fluid-filled, it develops an appearance similar to the ventricles. Intraparenchymal haemorrhage is characterised by an area of hyperattenuation (brightness) because congealed blood has a higher density than the surrounding brain tissue (*see* Figure 10.3).

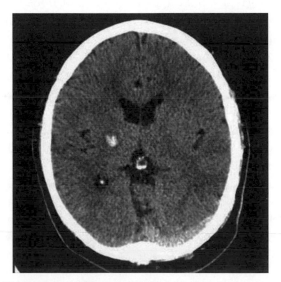

FIGURE 10.3 Small intracerebral haemorrhage in the right internal capsule

These appearances develop immediately, but with time, intracerebral haemorrhage becomes indistinguishable from areas of established cerebral infarction. A NCCT scan is also a sensitive and specific test for early subarachnoid haemorrhage where congealed blood is seen as hyperintensity within the subarachnoid space. A NCCT also allows detection of important complications of acute stroke, such as cerebral oedema and hydrocephalus.

CONTRAST-ENHANCED CT SCANNING

The diagnostic utility of CT scanning can be enhanced by the use of intravenous contrast agents that allow blood within blood vessels to be visualized and the passage of contrast through the brain to be monitored. This aids detection of highly vascular lesions such as arteriovenous malformations or tumours, but more importantly, contrast techniques allow CT angiography and CT perfusion images to be generated.

CT angiography involves intravenous injection of contrast medium and rapid acquisition of images from the aortic arch to the Circle of Willis. The dense contrast medium highlights blood vessels, allowing detection of arterial thrombotic occlusion or stenosis (including carotid artery stenosis). Arterial occlusion may thus be demonstrated even when NCCT of brain parenchyma appears normal. Asymmetry of contrast distribution can be seen in an area of ischaemia during conduct of a CT angiogram, and this principle forms the basis of CT perfusion imaging. A CT angiography image is shown in Figure 10.4.

CT perfusion involves repeated scanning of an area of brain as a bolus of intravenous contrast passes through it. This is either done at a single location, such as the level of the basal ganglia, but can be done in contiguous regions but currently only in thicker slice increments than a NCCT. It therefore has limited utility in the evaluation of acute brainstem or small volume ischaemia and is of most use in larger volume cortical and subcortical ischaemia. It allows measurement of cerebral blood flow and cerebral blood volume and other parameters such as time to peak and mean transit time. Time to peak is defined as the time taken for peak contrast enhancement in a region of brain tissue. Mean transit time is the mean time taken for contrast to perfuse an area of brain tissue. These measures can be compared between different regions of brain and thus aid rapid detection of ischaemia. Further, there is some evidence that these parameters can be used to predict whether areas of ischaemic brain can survive. For example, in an area of ischaemia, cerebral blood flow will be reduced and mean transit time and time to peak will be increased. Cerebral blood volume may also be increased, and if so, this is felt to signify irreversible ischaemia and impending infarction. An ischaemic area with reduced cerebral blood flow and increased transit time but preserved cerebral blood volume may signify salvageable tissue and is often referred to as a cerebral blood flow to blood volume mismatch.

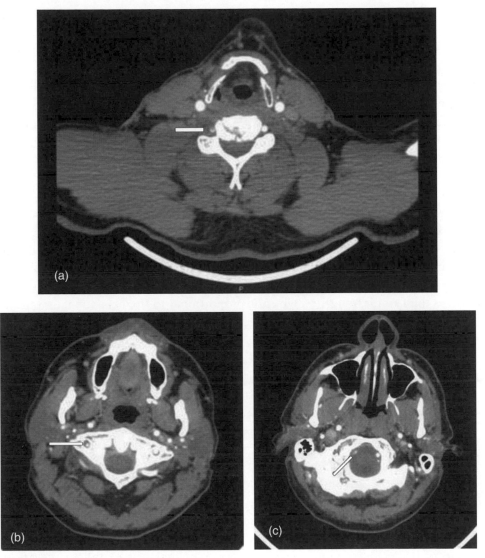

FIGURE 10.4 CT angiography image from a man with a right vertebral artery dissection. The relatively narrow lumen can clearly be seen throughout the entire length of the right vertebral artery

BASIC PRINCIPLES OF MAGNETIC RESONANCE IMAGING

The underlying principles of magnetic resonance imaging are complex and a detailed understanding is generally not required. MRI provides greater information than CT imaging in the context of acute stroke. For example, it is now possible to identify ischaemic brain tissue within minutes of symptom onset and it provides greater diagnostic certainty when there has been a significant delay to presentation.

Tissues of the human body are largely composed of water molecules and fat. Both contain hydrogen atoms, and it is the behaviour of hydrogen nuclei when exposed to a magnetic field that is exploited in brain MR imaging. An electrically neutral hydrogen atom consists of a single proton and a single electron. These protons spin around their own axes, producing a small magnetic field or a magnetic moment. In the body, these magnetic fields are arranged in such a way that there is no overall magnetic field. However, this changes when the atoms are placed in a magnetic field, or for our purposes, when a patient's body is placed inside an MR scanner.

When protons are exposed to a strong magnetic field, they align with the magnetic field with a small majority in the parallel state (a low-energy state in the direction of the magnetic field) and the remainder in a higher-energy anti-parallel state, or in opposition to the magnetic field. This is often referred to as net magnetization in the direction of the main magnetic field. When aligned, the protons precess, which means they deviate slightly in the direction they face, a little like a spinning top. This occurs at a frequency described by the Larmor equation, termed the Larmor frequency, which is proportional to the field strength and the magnetogyric ratio. This frequency is called the radio frequency range, and if a second magnetic pulse is sent with this frequency, those protons will respond by absorbing energy and the direction of the net magnetisation can be rotated by 90 degrees. This is known as excitation and yields protons that are all in a higher-energy state. It is also important to note that in this state, the protons spin (or precess) in the same phase, as if all the spinning tops were set off at the same time. This is not normally the case. Once this second radio frequency pulse is turned off, the protons will recover to the normal alignment or equilibrium state (the initial magnetised state as they are still under the influence of the first magnetic field). It is the properties of this relaxation phase that are crucial in the generation of clinical images as they differ depending on the environment in which the protons are bound—essentially the body tissue in which they are found. The difference is most apparent between fat and water molecules but occurs between other tissues. There are two main components to this relaxation, known as T1 and T2 relaxation. T1 relaxation refers to the release of absorbed energy by the excited protons and occurs at a different rate in different tissues. T2 relaxation refers to the process by which the excited protons begin to spin out of phase and is again dependent upon the environment in which the proton is found. The release of this absorbed energy can be detected by the receive coil in the scanner and thus differences between adjacent tissues can be defined.

MRI scans employ different sequences that are defined sets of magnetic pulses utilised to tease out differences and increase image contrast between body tissues. Sequences can also be T1- or T2-weighted and the key sequences used in evaluation of acute stroke are shown in Table 10.1. In general, bone, air, and CSF appear dark on T1-weighted images. In T2 sequences, bone and air appear dark but CSF and

TABLE 10.1 Summary of key imaging modalities and findings in acute stroke

Imaging modality—MRI

T1-weighted image	CSF has low-signal intensity compared to brain tissue
T2-weighted image	Bone and air appear dark but CSF and fatty tissues appear bright
Diffusion-weighted imaging	Areas of infarction appear bright but have reduced signal on the apparent diffusion coefficient map
Perfusion-weighted imaging	Colour maps of cerebral blood volume, cerebral blood flow, mean transit time, and time to peak are created
Cerebral infarction	Appears bright on diffusion-weighted image but dark on T1-weighted images and bright on T2-weighted images
Imaging modality—CT	
Cerebral infarction	Appears as area of hypoattenuation, although early signs may be subtle
Cerebral haemorrhage	Appears as area of hyperattenuation but ultimately after a prolonged period as an area of hypoattenuation
Perfusion imaging	Colour maps of cerebral blood volume, cerebral blood flow, mean transit time, and time to peak are created

fatty tissues appear bright, except in a T2-weighted FLAIR (fluid attenuation inversion recovery) image, where the signal from fluid (CSF) is suppressed, which gives greater signal contrast to detect small periventricular lesions. An infarct, or area of cytotoxic oedema, will appear dark on a T1 image and bright on a T2 image, while a haemorrhage will appear bright on both. Gradient echo sequences further aid the distinction between infarction and haemorrhage, although in general terms, this requires greater skill and experience than with CT scanning. The changes of acute infarction usually appear earlier than with CT and are detected with greater sensitivity, but additional techniques are required to allow immediate rapid confirmation of cerebral ischaemia.

DIFFUSION-WEIGHTED IMAGING AND MR PERFUSION IMAGING

Diffusion-weighted (DW) imaging is the most sensitive sequence for detection of acute infarction and changes are apparent within 20 minutes after ictus, when appearances on CT imaging and standard MRI sequences are unchanged. As mentioned, acute infarction leads to the development of cytotoxic oedema and water accumulation in cells. There is thus less diffusion or so-called 'random Brownian motion' of water molecules in an area of infarction. The movement of water molecules under the influence of a magnetic field will also be different and it is this effect that is measured during DW-MRI. Such an area of restricted diffusion appears bright on a diffusion-weighted image, although there is an important caveat to this. Chronic T2 changes can lead to increased signal on a DW image and this is termed 'T2 shine through.' To distinguish this and confirm that the cerebral ischaemia is acute, apparent diffusion coefficient (ADC) maps are generated. These incorporate only diffusion data and are thus more specific but the diffusion abnormality appears darker, as an area of reduced signal. A typical DWI study will incorporate three sequences, an e0 sequence that is in essence a T2-weighted signal that will be susceptible to T2 shine through, and an e500 signal and e1000 sequence, which are less susceptible and better able to confirm acute ischaemia. An example of a diffusion-weighted image is shown in Figure 10.5.

Perfusion-weighted MRI is similar in principle to CT perfusion. Rapid image acquisition following a bolus of intravenous contrast is performed and maps of cerebral blood volume, cerebral blood flow, and mean transit time are created. The advantage of MR perfusion is that the perfusion abnormality can be interpreted in light of the known diffusion abnormality. The diffusion abnormality is thought to represent irreversibly damaged brain tissue. The difference between the perfusion and diffusion image is termed the MR perfusion-diffusion mismatch and represents potentially salvageable tissue. MR angiography is again similar in principle to CT angiography and harnesses the different properties of flowing blood compared to its surrounding tissues to provide images of blood vessel anatomy and thereby detect vessel stenosis and occlusion. It can be done without use of contrast but contrast-enhanced MRA is superior.

WHAT TO USE: MRI OR CT?

There are some important practical issues that will become less important as technology advances. Scanning times are longer with MRI than with CT imaging and the noise and small bore of the scanner mean many patients fail to tolerate it. Further, because of the strong magnetic field generated during scanning, no ferrous material can be brought into the scanning room. This includes most resuscitation equipment and implantable metallic devices, meaning some patients simply cannot undergo MRI scanning. However, MRI has several advantages. It affords superior image quality for posterior fossa structures, allows rapid detection of acute infarction, provides better distinction between more recent and old areas of cerebral infarction, and shows a better distinction between areas of old cerebral infarction and haemorrhage. Importantly, this is with similar sensitivity for detection of intracerebral haemorrhage in the acute setting. MRI is thus the investigation of choice if it is available and tolerated by the patient.

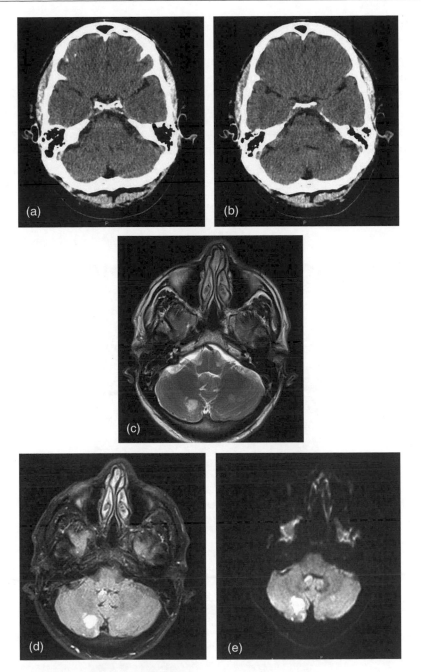

FIGURE 10.5 CT and MRI images from a man with a right vertebral artery dissection. His initial non-contrast CT scan, performed at the same time as the CT angiogram shown in Figure 10.4, was normal (top panel). A few days later, cerebellar infarction was evident on the T2-weighted image (middle panel), the T2 FLAIR image (bottom left panel), and the diffusion-weighted image (bottom right panel). The diffusion-weighted image would have revealed infarction at the time of the initial CT scan

CAROTID ARTERY IMAGING

Early assessment of the internal carotid artery is imperative in those with anterior circulation stroke. If a stenosis is found on the ipsilateral side, this represents an important opportunity to minimise risk of a further event. The three methods in routine clinical use are Doppler ultrasound, CT angiography, and MR angiography, with or without contrast. All modalities have high sensitivity for severe (70 to 99% stenosis) but ultrasound is less specific for the severity of stenosis and does not provide information on structure of other extracranial and intracranial arteries. As a result, if ultrasound is the initial imaging modality and is abnormal and suggests a greater than 50% stenosis, a second corroborative type of scan is required before proceeding to carotid surgery.

Images from a normal carotid ultrasound scan are shown in Figure 10.6. The normal flow velocity in the internal carotid artery is < 125 cm/s. The stenosis may

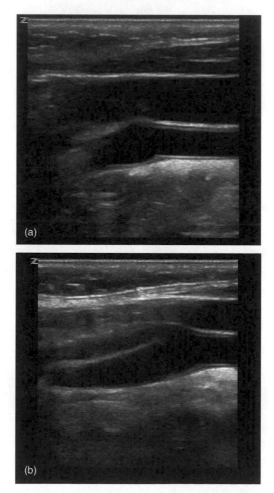

FIGURE 10.6 Carotid artery ultrasound image. The left common carotid artery and carotid bulb are shown in the top panel and the left internal carotid artery is shown in the bottom panel

be visualised on ultrasound, although often the spatial resolution is insufficient and flow velocity measures are used to confirm the presence and degree of stenosis. Flow velocity rises in the presence of carotid stenosis, and velocity above 125 cm/s is used to signify the presence of stenosis. A flow velocity of > 230 cm/s is typically used to signify a ≥ 70% carotid stenosis. It is important to note that in near complete occlusion, the velocity begins to fall and Doppler imaging could thus yield a false negative result.

TRANSCRANIAL DOPPLER IMAGING

Ultrasound waves are attenuated by bone, meaning conventional structural ultrasound imaging of the brain is not possible. However, the use of low-frequency ultrasound does allow ultrasound waves to penetrate the brain. The spatial resolution is poor but the Doppler effect can be measured. Essentially, ultrasound waves pass through the skull and if directed toward a major blood vessel, are deflected back by circulating blood elements (predominantly red blood cells) and thus measurement of flow velocity, direction of flow, and detection of flow artefact is possible. Transcranial Doppler (TCD) is portable and can be performed at the bedside, providing a means of continuous monitoring in those with acute stroke. The potential for use of TCD to improve outcomes in those treated with thrombolysis for acute ischaemic stroke is dealt with elsewhere.

TCD is performed using 2-Mhz ultrasound equipment and a small probe. A fixation device can be used to facilitate continuous imaging. The middle, anterior, and posterior cerebral segments of the internal carotid arteries are imaged through the temporal window located just above the zygomatic arch. The ophthalmic artery and internal carotid artery siphon can be visualized through the ophthalmic window and the vertebral arteries and basilar arteries can be seen via the foraminal window. A low power setting must be used for ophthalmic window insonation.

A standard diagnostic TCD examination begins with identification of the temporal insonation window, which is unfortunately absent in approximately 10% of cases. Blood flow should then be identified in each major branch of the Circle of Willis and information regarding the flow velocity and waveform characteristics recorded. Following this, the ophthalmic artery and internal carotid artery siphon are visualized via the ophthalmic window and then the basilar and vertebral arteries are visualized via the foraminal window. The key characteristics of each vessel are shown in Table 10.2. An example of a normal TCD trace is shown in Figure 10.7 (*see* plate section).

Detection of arterial occlusion and stenosis

These will be discovered during a standard diagnostic examination. Arterial occlusion or stenosis will cause a change in the flow velocity and/or the waveform

TABLE 10.2 Key characteristics of major vessels on transcranial Doppler imaging

Vessel	Insonation window	Depth	Flow direction	Flow velocity
MCA	Temporal	45–55 mm	Toward	30–80 cm/s
ACA	Temporal	60–75 mm	Away	30–80 cm/s
C1 ICA	Temporal	60–70 mm	Toward	30–80 cm/s
PCA	Temporal	55–75 mm	Toward/Away	20–60 cm/s
Ophthalmic	Ophthalmic	40–50 mm	Toward	Variable
ICA Siphon	Ophthalmic	55–65 mm	Toward/Away	20–70 cm/s
Vertebral	Foraminal	40–75 mm	Away*	20–50 cm/s
Basilar	Foraminal	75–110 mm	Away	20–60 cm/s

*Flow toward the probe may be seen from cerebellar arteries on transforaminal imaging.
MCA = middle cerebral artery, ACA = anterior cerebral artery, PCA = posterior cerebral artery and
ICA = internal carotid artery

characteristics. For example, in complete occlusion, flow will be absent with an altered flow pattern proximally. Flow velocity across a stenosis is increased, whereas in near occlusion, the waveform will be abnormal and have a high resistance pattern.

The degree of arterial occlusion in acute stroke can be estimated by the thrombolysis in brain ischemia (TIBI) grades, which help facilitate diagnosis but also allow monitoring of thrombolytic therapy. For example, the process of recanalzation can be monitored, and when this occurs, the odds of a favourable outcome are increased.

Microemboli detection

Asymptomatic microembolic signals (MES) can be detected using TCD and should be looked for in all individuals with carotid stenosis. They are thought to represent thrombi and platelet fibrin aggregates and are found in those with carotid artery disease. They are more common in those with recent symptoms and in those with atrial fibrillation and they arise during cardiac and aortic surgery and can be found thereafter in those with cardiac valve prostheses, particularly metallic valves. In those with recently symptomatic carotid stenosis, they are seen in approximately 40% of individuals and predict increased stroke risk. The increase in risk may be as high as eightfold in those with carotid disease and microemboli compared to carotid disease alone, although the true magnitude of this risk is unclear.

They are detected on TCD imaging because circulating emboli cause turbulence of blood flow and subsequent signal artefact, which is both visible and audible. They must be differentiated from other sources of artefact such as movement but this is usually (but not always) easy in practice. Patients with microemboli should be considered for carotid endarterectomy like all those with symptomatic carotid stenosis and there is some evidence that aggressive antiplatelet therapy reduces excess stroke risk. MES frequency is reduced by aspirin, but more marked effects are seen with the addition of clopidogrel and with the platelet glycoprotein inhibitor tirofibran. The use of clopidogrel for example is unlicensed in this setting but is used by many.

Assessment of cerebrovascular reactivity

TCD can be used to measure cerebral vasomotor reactivity (CVR), which is the compensatory dilatatory capacity of cerebral resistance vessels in response to increased arterial carbon dioxide concentration. In clinical practice, this response is manipulated by breath hold or infusion of acetazolamide. This should cause an increase in blood flow, which manifests as an increase in the flow velocity in the middle cerebral artery. The magnitude of this velocity change is a measure of CVR. Impaired CVR is a potential pathogenic mechanism in lacunar cerebral infarction but its main clinical application is in those with carotid artery stenosis. Distal to a stenosis, arteries will dilate in an attempt to maintain forward blood flow, and in some cases, the small resistance vessels dilate to their maximal capacity. In this situation, no further dilatation in response to increased carbon dioxide concentration can occur. TCD-measured flow velocity will therefore not increase as normal. This finding is associated with increased risk of stroke in those with carotid disease.

TCD bubble test

A TCD bubble test is a screening test for a right-to-left shunt. To perform the test, a venflon is inserted into an antecubital vein of a supine patient. The middle cerebral artery is insonated and the patient is injected with contrast media. Agitated saline is the contrast medium of choice and is prepared using 9 ml of normal saline and 1 ml of air that is mixed (thereby creating microbubbles) via a three-way stopcock and injected as a bolus. In the normal situation, these microbubbles enter the pulmonary circulation and are filtered by the lungs. In the presence of a right-to-left shunt, such as a PFO, septal defect, or intrapulmonary shunt, these microbubbles enter the systemic circulation and some enter the cerebral circulation. These microbubbles cause signal artefact on the TCD spectral signal. The test is then repeated during a Valsalva manouvre, which provides greater sensitivity by increasing the likelihood of a right-to-left shunt. If no microbubbles are seen, the test is negative and a clinically significant PFO is unlikely to be present. If a 'curtain sign' is found (where the spectral signal is almost entirely replaced by artifact), then a right-to-left shunt is confirmed and further assessment is warranted. The significance of a small number of microbubbles is less clear, but in the context of cryptogenic stroke should prompt further evaluation.

Transoesophageal echocardiography is the gold standard investigation for detection of a cardiac right-to-left shunt. Sensitivity can be improved by use of contrast media, and although sensitivity is similar to TCD-based assessment, it is more specific as it allows direct visualisation of the atrial septum and distinction between PFO and other cardiac defects. In some cases, transthoracic echocardiography provides diagnostic clarity but its sensitivity is less. The disadvantages of transoesophageal echocardiography are that it is associated with a small but important risk and requires sedation and participants cannot perform Valsalva manoeuvres during the test.

CHAPTER 11

Future directions in stroke treatment

INTRODUCTION

Despite the concerted efforts of scientists and clinical investigators worldwide, there are only a few acute strategies proven to improve outcome after stroke, and strategies to prevent stroke remain limited, as evidenced by the high rates of recurrent stroke seen in clinical trials. Current management of stroke is discussed in Chapter 6. This final chapter will review a number of strategies that are currently being evaluated as potential future treatments.

ACUTE STRATEGIES

Early 'neuroprotection'

The goal of these strategies is to maintain tissue viability in the very early phase of ischaemic stroke with a view to increasing the tissue that can be salvaged once reperfusion occurs. The ideal agent for this purpose would be easy to administer (ideally by paramedics in a pre-hospital setting) and have a low toxicity profile, as patients with stroke mimics would inevitably be treated on occasion. No such treatment exists at present, although intravenous magnesium sulphate has shown some promise in this context and remains under evaluation. Magnesium slows neuronal calcium influx (a process involved in the ischaemic cascade that culminates in cell death) and may induce local cerebral microcirculatory changes after ischaemic stroke. It is generally well tolerated and has been used in the management of pre-eclampsia for many years. Following some encouraging pilot studies, a phase 3 trial of pre-hospital magnesium treatment is underway.[1]

Other pharmacological techniques include free-radical scavenging agents, designed to 'mop up' the small, highly reactive 'free radical' compounds released by ischaemic tissue. These free radicals are thought to augment ischaemic damage though deleterious interactions with membranes of adjacent cells. This approach is appealing as free radical release is a final common pathway in the complex biochemical cascade that occurs after stroke, and reducing their effect may have greater influence than strategies that target specific processes earlier in the cascade. Clinical endpoint studies of free radical scavenging compounds have been negative thus far;[2–4] however, work continues in this area.

Induction of hypothermia slows tissue metabolism and in experimental models of stroke is effective in protecting the brain from ischaemic damage. Translation of experimental success into clinical management of stroke patients is challenging; however, a variety of cooling strategies for stroke patients have been developed, ranging from chilled bedding materials through to intravascular heat-exchange devices. Induction of moderate hypothermia appears to be feasible;[5, 6] however, at present there is insufficient data to justify its use in routine management of stroke.

Augmentation of cerebral perfusion

Angiographic studies in acute stroke suggest that the presence of good collateral blood flow is a determinant of outcome. Diversion of blood to the cerebral vasculature may enhance endogenous compensatory mechanisms and reduce infarction. Mechanical approaches to the augmentation of cerebral blood flow after stroke have been developed and are being evaluated: these may be invasive, such as the NeuroFlo device,[7] which, when inserted percutaneously to the descending aorta, partially occludes this vessel and enhances cerebral blood flow by diverting cardiac output from the lower extremities. A large phase 3 trial of the NeuroFlo device has recently completed recruitment although no efficacy data is yet available. An alternative approach that remains under evaluation uses inflatable cuffs that compress the limbs during the cardiac cycle and divert blood from the peripheries to the cerebral circulation.

Improving thrombolysis

Extending the time window

When administered intravenously within 4.5 hours of symptom onset, thrombolytic therapy with recombinant tissue plasminogen activator (rt-PA) improves outcome and is the most effective acute strategy in the management of ischaemic stroke. At present, only a minority of stroke patients receive this treatment, largely because the time taken to recognise symptoms, seek help, reach an appropriate facility, and complete the necessary investigations exceeds the time window within which the treatment must be delivered. Extension of the time window would increase number of patients eligible to receive this treatment and the third International Stroke Trial (IST3)[8] will address whether the standard dose of rt-PA remains safe and effective up to six hours after symptom onset.

Preclinical evidence suggests a differential safety and efficacy profile of alternate thrombolytic agents, and among these, desmoteplase (a highly fibrin-specific thrombolytic agent originally isolated from the saliva of the vampire bat) has undergone extensive evaluation in stroke patients using a longer time window.[9-11] A large trial of this agent in highly selected patients within nine hours of hemispheric stroke is underway.

Advances in brain imaging may have a role in improving selection of those patients most likely to benefit from lytic therapy. It is probable that some patients presenting outwith current time windows for thrombolysis still have salvageable brain tissue and may benefit from lysis. A growing body of evidence suggests that these patients may be identified with brain imaging. Perfusion studies (with CT or MRI) may identify tissue that is outwith the ischaemic core but threatened by hypoperfusion and potentially salvageable with lysis. Several clinical studies[12, 13] have sought to explore the potential benefit of treatment outwith conventional time windows in those with evidence of persisting penumbra, and some have suggested an association between early reperfusion and improved outcome. These early studies in stroke patients have enhanced our understanding of the evolution of acute stroke, and in the future, protocols for use of lytic therapy may be altered to accommodate more sophisticated imaging as our knowledge grows.

Augmenting pharmacological clot lysis
Mechanical clot disruption

Pharmacological thrombolysis is associated with systemic and intracranial bleeding complications (*see* Chapter 7), and rates of recanalisation are variable, particularly in the context of large clot-occluding proximal intracranial vessels. Mechanical thromboembolectomy offers a more direct means of disrupting and extracting such clots, with potential for more timely restoration of blood flow. A number of devices have been developed and some have been approved for use in selected patients with stroke; however, none is commonly used in the UK. The MERCI retriever is among the best-known device: this is a percutaneous catheter-mounted snare that allows the clot to be withdrawn into a more proximal catheter and then removed: recanalisation rates of 68% have been reported when this device is used as an adjunct to thrombolytic therapy.[14] Other devices currently under evaluation employ microcatheter manipulations, stenting (with and without adjuvant GPIIb/IIIa inhibitors), and intra-arterial ultrasound.[15-17]

Ultrasound

Preclinical studies suggest that fibrinolysis may be enhanced by exposure of a clot to ultrasound. Energy imparted to the clot (in the form of pressure waves) disrupts its structure and improves the penetration of thrombolytic agent, accelerating its destruction. The potential benefit of ultrasound (either transcranial or intra-arterial by means of a transducer placed on the tip of a catheter) has been examined in a series of small clinical trials.[18] Early evidence is encouraging and justifies further work in this area, although the routine combination of ultrasound and pharmacological lysis is not currently supported. There is some early evidence that the co-administration of microbubbles with ultrasound enhances clot disruption by increasing acoustic cavitation.[19] Further work to establish the potential role for sonothrombolysis in the management of stroke is underway.

SECONDARY PREVENTION
New drugs in the prevention of stroke
Novel oral anticoagulants

Antagonists of vitamin K such as warfarin have been used for decades in the management of many cardiovascular disorders, including stroke. The major factor limiting the use of warfarin is safety, as use of oral anticoagulants is associated with elevated risk of bleeding events, particularly in the context of overanticoagulation. This risk necessitates regular and careful monitoring of all patients taking warfarin or equivalent drugs, with appropriate dose adjustment. Although advances in pharmacogenomics hold the potential to reduce the burden of monitoring to a degree (*see* below), the development of novel antithrombotic agents that do not require such monitoring has been a major focus of research activity in recent years.

Novel oral anticoagulants that inhibit factor Xa (rivaroxaban) and IIa (dabigatran) have recently been developed. In clinical trials, these agents have shown promise in a variety of prothrombotic conditions. Of particular relevance to cerebrovascular medicine is the RELY study 20, which demonstrated non-inferiority of dabigatran to warfarin in the prevention of stroke related to atrial fibrillation. In this study, the recipients of dabigatran at a dose of 150 mg per day had a lower rate of stroke and similar rate of bleeding complications as those patients taking warfarin. Dabigatran confers the additional advantage of being a fixed-dose agent with no need for regular monitoring and fewer interactions with food and other drugs. These advantages come at a cost, however, as dabigatran is significantly more expensive to provide than warfarin.

Pharmacogenomics of secondary prevention strategies

With the elucidation of the human genome sequence over the past decade, pharmacogenomics has rapidly evolved into an important area of stroke medicine research. Pharmacogenomics studies the variability in drug response between different patient genotypes.[21] This altered drug activity could potentially result in reduced drug efficacy or adverse drug reactions (ADRs). Current translational research is focusing on testing patient genetic profiles and utilising this genomic information to provide more effective targeting of drug therapy in clinical practice.[22, 23] There has been considerable interest in the role of warfarin and clopidogrel pharmacogenomics, in optimising secondary vascular disease preventative therapy, and in minimising the risk of haemorrhagic complications.[24, 25]

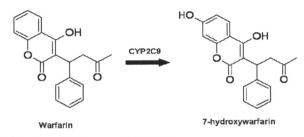

FIGURE 11.1 Warfarin metabolism and CYP2C9

Warfarin is metabolised by the cytochrome P450 2C9 enzyme (CYP2C9) into its major inactive metabolite, 7-hydroxywarfarin (*see* Figure 11.1).[26] Genome-wide association studies (GWAS) have identified genetic polymorphisms of CYP2C9 as an important determinant of warfarin activity.[27] The two common allelic variants, CYP2C9*2 and CYP2C9*3, result in poor metaboliser (PM) phenotypes and display reduced warfarin metabolism.[28] These patients' genotypes have been shown to have an increased risk of overcoagulation and haemorrhagic complications.[29, 30] The therapeutic target for warfarin, Vitamin K epoxide reductase complex 1 (VKORC1), also displays genetic polymorphism and pharmacogenetic variability.[27, 31] These mutations have been associated with both warfarin resistance and increased drug sensitivity.[32] There has therefore been increasing interest in the role of genotype-guided warfarin therapy in clinical practice.[33] The FDA approved warfarin genotype-testing in 2007 and has recently updated its label for warfarin pharmacogenetic testing (www.pharmgkb.org/clinical/warfarin.jsp). Various PCR-based genotyping methods are now available and some have been approved by the FDA.[34, 35]

Recent clinical studies have shown that genotype-guided warfarin dosing is more accurate in determining the initial loading doses, especially in patients requiring low- or high-dose maintenance warfarin therapy.[36, 37] Genotype-guided dosing has also been shown to achieve better anticoagulation control and less risk of ADRs.[38] However, results have been conflicting, with other clinical studies showing no benefit of genotype-guided warfarin therapy.[39, 40] Larger prospective warfarin clinical pharmacogenetic studies with more rigorous study design are ongoing.[41] The newer anticoagulant agents display little CYP enzyme metabolism and therefore avoid this pharmacogenetic variability in drug effect.[42, 43] The direct thrombin inhibitor, dabigatran etexilate, has shown promising results in reducing stroke risk in patients with AF and could supersede warfarin therapy in the future.[43]

Clopidogrel is being increasingly used in the treatment of acute coronary syndrome and in secondary stroke prevention therapy. One of its important treatment indications is in reducing the risk of coronary artery stent thrombosis, post-percutaneous coronary intervention (PCI). There has been major interest in the effect of CYP2C19 pharmacogenetics on the antiplatelet activity of clopidogrel.[44] Clopidogrel is a prodrug, which is metabolised by the CYP2C19 enzyme into its

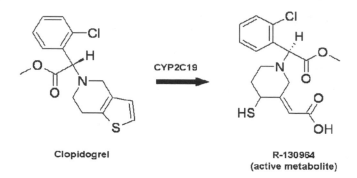

FIGURE 11.2 Clopidogrel metabolism and CYP2C19

active metabolite (*see* Figure 11.2). This irreversibly inhibits the P2Y12 receptor on the platelet surface, which subsequently blocks the activation of the GpIIb/IIIa pathway that is associated with the cross-linking of platelets via fibrin.[45] Drugs that inhibit CYP2C19 enzyme function have been shown to reduce clopidogrel activation. Some commonly used proton pump inhibitors have been associated with reduced clopidogrel efficacy, and current clinical guidelines recommend avoiding these drug combinations.[46, 47]

CYP2C19 genetic polymorphism has been shown to affect clopidogrel antiplatelet activity. CYP2C19*2 and CYP2C19*3 are the most common allelic variants, which both result in PM phenotypes.[48] CYP2C19 PMs have displayed higher plasma clopidogrel concentrations and lower antiplatelet effects compared to extensive metabolisers.[49] Patients with low CYP2C19 enzyme activity have been shown to have increased risk of cardiovascular events and coronary stent thrombosis.[50] CYP2C19*17 is a newly identified allelic variant, which is associated with a specific promoter polymorphism that results in increased enzyme metabolic activity.[51] Increased activation of clopidogrel in patients with the CYP2C19*17 genotype has been shown to increase the risk of bleeding.[52] Further analysis of these CYP2C19 genetic polymorphisms and their pharmacogenetic effects are ongoing.[53] The FDA has recently updated its label for clopidogrel pharmacogenetic testing (www. pharmgkb.org/clinical/clopidogrel.jsp).

There has also been increasing interest in the role of platelet function testing in guiding clopidogrel therapy.[54] Various platelet function assays are being researched into assessing the pharmacodynamic effects of clopidogrel.[55] Clinical studies have demonstrated that platelet aggregation studies could potentially be used to reduce clopidogrel-related bleeding complications.[56] The role of platelet function testing in optimising clopidogrel treatment in post-PCI and coronary artery stenting is currently being investigated in a large multi-centre clinical trial.[57] Combined pharmacogenetic and pharmacodynamic testing to optimise clopidogrel antiplatelet activity may be the best approach in secondary vascular disease preventative strategies in the future.[58] Current clinical guidelines recommend using higher doses of clopidogrel in patients showing low antiplatelet activity or switching to the newer, more potent P2Y12 inhibitor prasugrel.[57, 58] However, prasugrel is contraindicated in stroke and elderly patients due to its higher risk of bleeding.

Pharmacogenomics represents an exciting area of personalised medicine research, with genotype-guided antithrombotic therapy having a potential role in optimising therapeutic efficacy in stroke patients. Despite these important advances in pharmacogenomics, translating these research findings into clinical practice remains a challenge. A more rigorous evidence base from larger pharmacogenomic clinical studies is required to aid development of clinical guidelines for appropriate use of these genotype tests.[59] Well-developed genomic services are also needed for effective implementation of genotype testing.[60] This will require education of healthcare staff in both the ethical and scientific aspects of pharmacogenomics. With current financial restrictions to healthcare budgets, funding these services will also be challenging.[61] However, with ongoing advances in genomic and translational medicine, genotype-guided therapies, and platelet function testing are likely to have some role in stroke treatment strategies in the near future.[62]

Warfarin is hydroxylated by CYP2C9 into the inactive metabolite 7-hydroxywarfarin. Patients with CYP2C9 poor metaboliser genotypes have an enhanced anticoagulation effect and an increased risk of haemorrhagic complications.

Clopidogrel is a prodrug, which is metabolised by CYP2C19 into its active metabolite that inhibits the P2Y12 platelet receptor. Poor metaboliser genotypes have demonstrated a reduced antiplatelet effect, whereas ultra-rapid metabolisers have a higher risk of bleeding.

REFERENCES

1. Saver JL, Kidwell C, Eckstein M, *et al.* Prehospital neuroprotective therapy for acutestroke results of the field administration of stroke therapy-magnesium (FAST-MAG) pilot trial. *Stroke.* 2004; **35**: e106–8.
2. Grotta J. Combination therapy with lubeluzole and t-PA in the treatment of acute ischemic stroke. Paper presented at: American Heart Association's 23rd International Joint Conference on Stroke; Anaheim, CA, 1998.
3. Bose A, Henkes H, Alfke K, *et al.* Penumbra Phase 1 Stroke Trial Investigators. The Penumbra System: a mechanical device for the treatment of acute stroke due to thromboembolism. *Am J Neuroradiol.* 2008; **29**: 1409–13.
4. Lees KR, Zivin JA, Ashwood T, *et al.* For the Stroke–Acute Ischemic NXY Treatment (SAINT I) Trial Investigators. NXY-059 for Acute Ischemic Stroke. *N Engl J Med.* 2006; **354**: 588–600.
5. Krieger DW, De Georgia MA, Abou-Chebl A, *et al.* Cooling for acute ischemic brain damage (COOL AID): an open pilot study of induced hypothermia in acute ischemic stroke. *Stroke.* 2001; **32**: 1847–54.
6. De Georgia MA, Krieger DW, Abou-Chebl A, *et al.* Cooling for acute ischemic brain damage (COOL AID): a feasibility trial of endovascular cooling. *Neurology.* 2004; **63**: 312–17.

7. Liebeskind DS. Aortic occlusion for cerebral ischemia: from theory to practice. *Curr Cardiol.* 2008; **10**: 31–6.

8. www.dcn.ed.ac.uk/ist3/

9. Hacke W, Albers G, Al-Rawi Y, *et al.* The desmoteplase in acute ischaemic stroke trial (DIAS). A phase II MRI-based 9-hour window acute stroke throbolysis trial with intravenous desmoteplase. *Stroke.* 2005; **36**: 66–73.

10. Furlan AJ, Eyding D, Albers GW, *et al.* Dose escalation of desmoteplase for acute ischaemic stroke (DEDAS): evidence of safety and efficacy 3 to 9 hours after stroke onset. *Stroke.* 2006; **37**: 1227–31.

11. Hacke W, Furlan AJ, Al-Rawi Y, *et al.* Intravenous desmoteplase in patients with acute ischaemic stroke selected by MRI perfusion-diffusion weighted imaging or perfusion CT (DIAS-2): a prospective, randomised, double-blind, placebo-controlled study. *Lancet Neurol.* 2009; **8**: 141–50.

12. Albers GW, Thijs VN, Wechsler L, *et al.* Magnetic resonance imaging profiles predict clinical response to early reperfusion: the diffusion and perfusion imaging evaluation for understanding stroke evolution (DEFUSE) study. *Ann Neurol.* 2006; **60**: 508–17.

13. Davis SM, Donnan GA, Parsons MW, *et al.* Effects of alteplase beyond 3h after stroke in the Echoplanar Imaging Thrombolytic Evaluation Trial (EPITHET): a placebo-controlled randomized trial. *Lancet Neurol.* 2008; **7**: 299–309.

14. Ringer AJ, Qureshi AI, Fessler RD, *et al.* Angioplasty of intracranial occlusion resistant to thrombolysis in acute ischemic stroke. *Neurosurgery.* 2001; **48**: 1282–90.

15. Smith WS, Sung G, Saver J, *et al.* Mechanical thrombectomy for acute ischemic stroke final results of the multi MERCI trial. *Stroke.* 2008; **39**: 1205–12.

16. Barnwell SL, Clark WM, Nguyen TT, *et al.* Safety and efficacy of delayed intraarterial urokinase therapy with mechanical clot disruption for thromboembolic stroke. *Am J Neuroradiol.* 1994; **15**: 1817–22.

17. Gobin YP, Starkman S, Duckwiler GR, *et al.* MERCI 1: a phase 1 study of mechanical embolus removal in cerebral ischemia. *Stroke.* 2004; **35**: 2848–54.

18. Alexandrov AV, Molina CA, Grotta JC, *et al.* Ultrasound-enhanced systemic thrombolysis for acute ischemic stroke. *N Engl J Med.* 2004; **351**: 2170–8.

19. Meairs S, Culp W. Microbubbles for thrombolysis of acute ischemic stroke. *Cerebrovasc Dis.* 2009; **27** (Suppl. 2): 55–65.

20. Connolly SJ, Ezekowitz, MD, Yusuf S, *et al.* Dabigatran versus warfarin in patients with atrial fibrillation. *N Engl J Med.* 2009; **361**: 1139–51.

21. Evans WE, McLeod HL. Pharmacogenomics: drug disposition, drug targets, and side effects. *N Engl J Med.* 2003; **348**(6): 538–49.

22. Feero WG, Guttmacher AE, Collins FS. Genomic medicine: an updated primer. *N Engl J Med.* 2010; **362**(21): 2001–11.

23. Hoffman EP. Skipping toward personalized molecular medicine. *N Engl J Med.* 2007; **357**(26): 2719–22.

24. Ashley EA, Butte AJ, Wheeler MT, *et al.* Clinical assessment incorporating a personal genome. *Lancet.* 2010; **375**(9725): 1525–35.

25. Schelleman H, Limdi NA, Kimmel SE. Ethnic differences in warfarin maintenance dose requirement and its relationship with genetics. *Pharmacogenomics.* 2008; **9**(9): 1331–46.

26. Kaminsky LS, Zhang ZY. Human P450 metabolism of warfarin. *Pharmacol Ther.* 1997; **73**(1): 67–74.

27. Cooper GM, Johnson JA, Langaee TY, *et al*. A genome-wide scan for common genetic variants with a large influence on warfarin maintenance dose. *Blood*. 2008; **112**(4): 1022–7.

28. Wadelius M, Pirmohamed M. Pharmacogenetics of warfarin: current status and future challenges. *Pharmacogenomics*. 2007; **7**(2): 99–111.

29. Higashi MK, Veenstra DL, Kondo LM, *et al*. Association between CYP2C9 genetic variants and anticoagulation-related outcomes during warfarin therapy. *JAMA*. 2002; **287**(13): 1690–8.

30. Lindh JD, Lundgren S, Holm L, *et al*. Several-fold increase in risk of overanticoagulation by CYP2C9 mutations. *Clin Pharmacol Ther*. 2005; **78**(5): 540–50.

31. Limdi NA, Beasley TM, Crowley MR, *et al*. VKORC1 polymorphisms, haplotypes and haplotype groups on warfarin dose among African-Americans and European-Americans. *Pharmacogenomics*. 2008; **9**(10): 1445–58.

32. Oldenburg J, Bevans CG, Fregin A, *et al*. Current pharmacogenetic developments in oral anticoagulation therapy: the influence of variant VKORC1 and CYP2C9 alleles. *Thromb Haemost*. 2007; **98**(3): 570–8.

33. Gage BF, Lesko LJ. Pharmacogenetics of warfarin: regulatory, scientific, and clinical issues. *J Thromb Thrombolysis*. 2008; **25**(1): 45–51.

34. King CR, Porche-Sorbet RM, Gage BF, *et al*. Performance of commercial platforms for rapid genotyping of polymorphisms affecting warfarin dose. *Am J Clin Pathol*. 2008; **129**(6): 876–83.

35. Langley MR, Booker JK, Evans JP, *et al*. Validation of clinical testing for warfarin sensitivity: comparison of CYP2C9-VKORC1 genotyping assays and warfarin-dosing algorithms. *J Mol Diagn*. 2009; **11**(3): 216–25.

36. The International Warfarin Pharmacogenetics Consortium. Estimation of the warfarin dose with clinical and pharmacogenetic data. *N Engl J Med*. 2009; **360**(8): 753–64.

37. Lenzini P, Wadelius M, Kimmel S, *et al*. Integration of genetic, clinical, and INR data to refine warfarin dosing. *Clin Pharmacol Ther*. 2010; **87**(5): 572–8.

38. Caraco Y, Blotnick S, Muszkat M. CYP2C9 genotype-guided warfarin prescribing enhances the efficacy and safety of anticoagulation: a prospective randomized controlled study. *Clin Pharmacol Ther*. 2008; **83**(3): 460–70.

39. Kangelaris KN, Bent S, Nussbaum RL, *et al*. Genetic testing before anticoagulation? A systematic review of pharmacogenetic dosing of warfarin. *J Gen Intern Med*. 2009; **24**(5): 656–64.

40. McMillin GA, Melis R, Wilson A, *et al*. Gene-based warfarin dosing compared with standard of care practices in an orthopedic surgery population: a prospective, parallel cohort study. *Ther Drug Monit*. 2010; **32**(3): 338–45.

41. van Schie RM, Wadelius MI, Kamali F, *et al*. Genotype-guided dosing of coumarin derivatives: the European pharmacogenetics of anticoagulant therapy (EU-PACT) trial design. *Pharmacogenomics*. 2009; **10**(10): 1687–95.

42. Samama MM, Gerotziafas GT. Newer anticoagulants in 2009. *J Thromb Thrombolysis*. 2010; **29**(1): 92–104.

43. Connolly SJ, Ezekowitz MD, Yusuf S, *et al*. Dabigatran versus warfarin in patients with atrial fibrillation. *N Engl J Med*. 2009; **361**(12): 1139–51.

44. Mega JL, Close SL, Wiviott SD, *et al*. Cytochrome p-450 polymorphisms and response to clopidogrel. *N Engl J Med*. 2009; **360**(4): 354–62.

45. Parikh SA, Beckman JA. Contemporary use of clopidogrel in patients with coronary artery disease. *Curr Cardiol Rep.* 2007; **9**(4): 257–63.
46. Cuisset T, Frere C, Quilici J, *et al.* Comparison of omeprazole and pantoprazole influence on a high 150-mg clopidogrel maintenance dose the PACA (Proton Pump Inhibitors And Clopidogrel Association) prospective randomized study. *J Am Coll Cardiol.* 2009; **54**(13): 1149–53.
47. Holmes DR, Jr, Dehmer GJ, Kaul S, *et al.* ACCF/AHA Clopidogrel clinical alert: approaches to the FDA 'boxed warning': a report of the American College of Cardiology Foundation Task Force on Clinical Expert Consensus Documents and the American Heart Association. *Circulation.* 2010; **122**(5): 537–57.
48. Desta Z, Zhao X, Shin JG, *et al.* Clinical significance of the cytochrome P450 2C19 genetic polymorphism. *Clin Pharmacokinet.* 2002; **41**(12): 913–58.
49. Kim KA, Park PW, Hong SJ, *et al.* The effect of CYP2C19 polymorphism on the pharmacokinetics and pharmacodynamics of clopidogrel: a possible mechanism for clopidogrel resistance. *Clin Pharmacol Ther.* 2008; **84**(2): 236–42.
50. Shuldiner AR, O'Connell JR, Bliden KP, *et al.* Association of cytochrome P450 2C19 genotype with the antiplatelet effect and clinical efficacy of clopidogrel therapy. *JAMA.* 2009; **302**(8): 849–57.
51. Rudberg I, Mohebi B, Hermann M, *et al.* Impact of the ultrarapid CYP2C19*17 allele on serum concentration of escitalopram in psychiatric patients. *Clin Pharmacol Ther.* 2008; **83**(2): 322–7.
52. Sibbing D, Koch W, Gebhard D, *et al.* Cytochrome 2C19*17 allelic variant, platelet aggregation, bleeding events, and stent thrombosis in clopidogrel-treated patients with coronary stent placement. *Circulation.* 2010; **121**(4): 512–18.
53. Ragia G, Arvanitidis KI, Tavridou A, *et al.* Need for reassessment of reported CYP2C19 allele frequencies in various populations in view of CYP2C19*17 discovery: the case of Greece. *Pharmacogenomics.* 2009; **10**(1): 43–9.
54. Collet JP, Montalescot G. Platelet function testing and implications for clinical practice. *J Cardiovasc Pharmacol Ther.* 2009; **14**(3): 157–69.
55. Bouman HJ, Parlak E, van Werkum JW, *et al.* Which platelet function test is suitable to monitor clopidogrel responsiveness? A pharmacokinetic analysis on the active metabolite of clopidogrel. *J Thromb Haemost.* 2010; **8**(3): 482–8.
56. Sibbing D, Schulz S, Braun S, *et al.* Antiplatelet effects of clopidogrel and bleeding in patients undergoing coronary stent placement. *J Thromb Haemost.* 2010; **8**(2): 250–6.
57. Price MJ, Berger PB, Angiolillo DJ, *et al.* Evaluation of individualized clopidogrel therapy after drug-eluting stent implantation in patients with high residual platelet reactivity: design and rationale of the GRAVITAS trial. *Am Heart J.* 2009; **157**(5): 818–24.
58. Wallentin L. P2Y(12) inhibitors: differences in properties and mechanisms of action and potential consequences for clinical use. *Eur Heart J.* 2009; **30**(16): 1964–77.
59. Limdi NA, Veenstra DL. Expectations, validity, and reality in pharmacogenetics. *J Clin Epidemiol.* 2010; **63**(9): 960–9.
60. Ormond KE, Wheeler MT, Hudgins L, *et al.* Challenges in the clinical application of whole-genome sequencing. *Lancet.* 2010; **375**(9727): 1749–51.

61. Frueh FW. Real-world clinical effectiveness, regulatory transparency and payer coverage: three ingredients for translating pharmacogenomics into clinical practice. *Pharmacogenomics.* 2010; **11**(5): 657–60.
62. Seip RL, Duconge J, Ruano G. Implementing genotype-guided antithrombotic therapy. *Future Cardiol.* 2010; **6**(3): 409–24.

Index

Tables and figures are given in italics.